Reinhard Graf   Brennan Wilson

Sonography of the Infant Hip
and its Therapeutic Implications

ISBN 3-8261-0041-7

Reinhard Graf   Brennan Wilson

Sonography of the Infant Hip and its Therapeutic Implications

In collaboration with Peter Schuler and Harry Merk
With a contribution by Karl Schneider

With 141 Figures and 17 Tables

CHAPMAN & HALL
London · Glasgow · Weinheim · New York
Tokyo · Melbourne · Madras

Univ.-Professor Dr. med. Reinhard Graf
Allgemeines und Orthopädisches
Landeskrankenhaus Stolzalpe
A-8852 Stolzalpe
Austria

Dr. Brennan Wilson
Department of Radiology
Royal Manchester Children's Hospital,
Pendlebury
Manchester, M 27 4HA
Great Britain

Translated and revised by Dr. Brennan Wilson

Title of the German Edition:
Sonographie der Säuglingshüfte und therapeutische Konsequenzen – Ein Kompendium
4th revised edition, © Enke 1993
Bücherei des Orthopäden, Suppelement to "Zeitschrift für Orthopäden"
incorporating "Aktuelle Orthopädie"
Published by J. Krämer and K.-F. Schlegel

Book production: PRO EDIT GmbH, D-69126 Heidelberg
Typesetting and Printing: Druckerei Zechner, D-67346 Speyer
Bookbinding: J. Schäffer GmbH & Co. KG, D-67269 Grünstadt
Printed on acid-free paper

To my teacher,
Univ.-Prof. Dr. H. Buchner,
whom I hold in high esteem
R. G.

To my mother
for teaching me to read
and my father
for sending me to medical school
B. P. M. W.

Acknowledgements

My thanks are due to my co-authors P. Schuler, K. Schneider and H. Merk, for the data and pictorial material they have put at my disposal. My thanks and recognition go to Kurt Lecher for his collaboration over many years and for his collection of images. I also owe personal thanks to Brennan Wilson for translating and arranging the fourth German edition in the English language.

Anyone who believes that he has found a perfect method should stop and consider carefully whether part of his brain has not gone to sleep.

Henry Ford

The current issues in hip sonography have changed as the technique has become increasingly widespread. The method itself has been proved to be practicable, reproducible, and capable of being learned and taught, and interest has moved away from this area towards the clinical implications. As the method is not an end in itself and should not remain hidden in an ivory tower, it has become necessary to evaluate results and report both the clinical and therapeutic import of the method.

The technical section has been shortened and limited to the essentials, and should serve as an introduction for beginners. In the section concerned with method we have taken great care to strike the correct balance. On the one hand, it is necessary to present the theoretic principles in order that the practicalities may be better understood. On the other hand, a review such as this should also give practical guidance. Based on 14 years' experience in the training of colleagues on countless courses, this review should also act as a resource on such courses. For this reason, typical mistakes have also been included.

The statistical section aims to give a summary and overview of results without any claim to being comprehensive.

We have received many requests to include a chapter on determination of therapy under ultrasound control, and this now appears for the first time. This shows the direct connections between the sonographic findings and the therapeutic implications. Lessons learned from the statistics and the sonographic follow-up of therapy have without doubt contributed to the fact that Austria has become the first country in the world to institute a routine prophylactic screening programme in hip sonography. The much-cited 'cook-book' character of the text has been retained without significantly widening its scope.

The book suits modern demands, keeping the basis for learning the method. It should also serve as a concise reference work for experienced users. It is difficult to have regard for scientific method, brevity, relevance, detailed explanation where appropriate, and conciseness, all together; the authors hope that critics will be forgiving, as we are more at home in the operating theatre than the study.

Stolzalpe, Summer 1993 *Reinhard Graf*

Contents

1	**Ultrasound physics**	1
	Historical background	1
1.1	Physical basis	2
1.1.1	Basic concepts	2
1.1.2	The production of ultrasound waves	2
1.1.3	Refraction	3
1.1.4	Diffraction	3
1.1.5	Scatter	3
1.1.6	Absorption of ultrasound	4
1.1.7	Methods of image production	4
1.1.8	Artefacts	4
1.2	Biological effects and questions of safety	5
	Key points	5
2	**Ultrasound equipment**	7
2.1	Superiority of real-time linear array transducers	7
2.2	Relative merits of linear and sector scanners *by Karl Schneider*	7
2.2.1	Preliminary remarks	7
2.2.2	Finding the standard plane of section	8
2.2.3	Contact of the ultrasound probe	8
2.2.4	Effective size of the image	8
2.2.5	The near field	9
2.2.6	Artefacts	10
2.2.7	Literature	11
2.3	Instrument settings	11
2.3.1	The acoustic output control	11
2.3.2	The depth gain control	12
2.3.3	The contrast control	12
2.3.4	The focal depth	12
2.3.5	Pre- and post-processing	12
2.4	Choice of instrument	12
2.5	Documentation of the hip sonogram	13
2.5.1	Formal image criteria	13
2.6	Equipment for documentation	15
	Key points	16
3	**The infant hip: historical review of diagnostic modalities**	17
3.1	Clinical diagnosis	17
3.2	Plain radiography	17
3.3	Arthrography	17
3.4	Computed tomography and magnetic resonance imaging (MRI)	18
	Key points	18
4	**Development, anatomy and pathological anatomy**	19
4.1	Development and anatomy	19
4.1.1	The femoral neck and head	19
4.1.2	The acetabulum	20
4.2	Morbid anatomy	21
4.2.1	Morphology and morphological changes in the pelvis following dislocation	21
4.2.2	Histological changes in the acetabulum in dislocation	23
	Key points	25
5	**Sonographic morphology of the infant hip**	27
5.1	The superficial soft tissues	27
5.2	The proximal end of the femur	28
5.2.1	The osteochondral junction	29
5.2.2	The connective tissue (capsular) fold	31
5.2.3	The femoral capital ossification centre	31
5.3	The acetabular roof	32
5.3.1	The parts of the acetabular roof	32

5.3.2   The perichondrium   33
5.3.3   The acetabular labrum   34
5.3.4   Questions of sonographic
        nomenclature   34
5.4   The floor of the acetabulum   .   35
5.4.1   The so-called 'fluid film'   35
5.4.2   The ligament of
        the head of the femur   36
5.5   Identification of anatomy
        at ultrasound:
        the standard situation   36
5.6   Practical procedure
        in difficult cases   37
5.6.1   Identification of
        the circumference
        of the femoral head   37
5.6.2   Misidentification of the bony
        rim and acetabular labrum   . .   37
        Key points   38

6   Sonographic typing
        of hip joints   39
6.1   Dividing hip joints
        into sonographic types   39
6.1.1   Type I   39
6.1.2   Type II   40
6.1.3   Type III   41
6.1.4   Type IV   46
6.1.5   Sonographic differentiation
        between types III and IV   . . .   47
6.2   The problem of the echogenic
        cartilaginous rim   48
6.2.1   The reference point   48
6.2.2   Reverberation artefacts   50
6.2.3   Pathological and
        physiological echogenicity   . .   50
        Key points   52

7   Standard levels,
        measurement technique
        and measurement errors   . .   53
7.1   The standard section   53
7.1.1   Variations in planes of section   .   53
7.2   The anatomical landmarks   . .   54
7.2.1   The inferior border of the iliac
        bone and the acetabular floor   .   54
7.2.2   The contour of the iliac wing   .   56
7.2.3   The acetabular labrum   57
7.3   Definition of the
        standard plane   57

7.4   Measurement techniques
        and mistakes of measurement   58
7.4.1   Introduction   58
7.4.2   The acetabular roof line   58
7.4.3   The base line   59
7.4.4   The cartilaginous roof line   . .   61
7.5   Comparison of
        ultrasound techniques   62
7.5.1   Advantages of
        the frontal approach   62
7.5.2   The 'internal approach'   63
7.5.3   The transverse approach   . . .   64
7.5.4   The posterior approach   64
7.5.5   The Lorenz position   64
7.5.6   The Harcke technique   64
        Key points   65

8   Determination of
        hip maturity with
        the sonometer   67
8.1   The sonometer   67
8.1.1   Historical note   68
8.2   Using the α and β angles to
        subdivide hip types   68
8.2.1   Types Ia and Ib   68
8.2.2   The causation of
        osteoarthrosis: a hypothesis   . .   71
8.2.3   The newborn hip joint: hips
        type IIa, IIa(+) and IIa(−)   .   71
8.2.4   Delay in ossification after
        the third month (type IIb)   . .   72
8.2.5   Classification
        of premature infants   73
8.2.6   The stability of hip joints:
        type IIc   73
8.2.7   Dislocated joints:
        types D, IIIa, IIIb, IV   74
        Key points   75

9   The stress or
        dynamic examination   77
9.1   Performing the
        dynamic examination   77
9.2   Natural elasticity
        of the hip joint   77
9.3   The unstable hip joint   77
9.4   The Ortolani phenomenon   . .   80
9.4.1   Tönnis's definition
        of the Ortolani sign   80
        Key points   81

**10   Reporting the
         hip sonogram** 83

10.1   Components of
         the sonogram report 83
10.1.1 Age of the patient 83
10.1.2 Description of the findings . . 83
10.1.3 Further definitions 83
10.1.4 Report on the angles 84
         Key points 85

**11   Positioning and
         manual technique** 87

11.1   General conduct
         of the examination 87
11.2   The cradle apparatus
         and positioning 87
11.3   Finger and hand position . . . 88
11.4   Manipulating the probe 91
         Key points 93

**12   Statistics, clinical findings
         and therapeutic
         implications** 95

12.1   Sonographic typing of hips . . 95
12.1.1 Frequency of pathological
         findings in high-risk groups . . 95
12.2   Historical risk factors
         and hip sonography 96
12.2.1 Breech presentation 96
12.2.2 Other anamnestic risk factors . 96
12.3   Clinical findings and
         hip sonography 97
12.3.1 Instability of the hip 97
12.3.2 Other clinical findings 98
12.4   Hip sonography
         and the radiograph 99
12.4.1 Are radiographs
         necessary at all? 99
12.4.2 The radiographic acetabular
         angle and the bony angle α
         on the sonogram 99
12.4.3 Tönnis's classification of
         subluxation and hip type . . . 100

12.5   Organisation of hip sonography
         and sonographic follow-up . . 101
12.5.1 The maturation curve 101
12.5.2 Neonatal screening 101
12.5.3 Follow-up intervals 102
12.5.4 Premature infants 102
         Key points 102

**13   Sonographic control
         of therapy** 103

13.1   Principles of treatment 103
13.2   Phases of treatment 103
13.2.1 Reduction phase 104
13.2.2 Retention phase 105
13.2.3 Late maturation phase 106
13.3   Problems in treatment 107
13.3.1 Exceptions in the case
         of neonates 107
13.3.2 Age limit 108
         Key points 108

**14   Sonographic follow-up:
         examples** 109

14.1   Hip joint type IIIa;
         progress under treatment . . . 109
14.2   Follow-up of progress patient
         W. D. Initial findings type IIIa 111
14.3   Follow-up for progress with
         conservative therapy
         (hip type D) 113
14.4   Follow-up for progress.
         Hip type IIIb with treatment
         in a Fettweis plaster 115
14.5   Follow-up for progress of
         type IIIb hip under therapy . . 115
14.6   Follow-up for progress
         in a type IIIa hip 119

**15   Examples for
         self assessment** 121

         Questions 121

         Subject Index 125

1 Ultrasound physics

Historical background

The existence of ultrasound was first suspected by the Italian researcher Ballanzani in the eighteenth century when he made his famous observation that bats could not orientate themselves in flight when their ears were stopped up. Ultrasound waves were first artificially produced in 1880 through the discovery of the so-called piezo-electric effect by the brothers J. and P. Curie. The first practical use of sonar was developed by A. Von Sternbert who was able to open it up to a wider maritime usage after the Titanic catastrophe in 1912.

In medicine, ultrasound diagnosis was first introduced into neurology by the neuro-

Table 1.1. Summary of literature in ultrasound of the musculoskeletal system

Kratochwil and Zweymüller	1974	Delineation of invasively growing bone tumours
Zweymüller et al.	1975	Localisation of psoas abscesses
Baumann and Kremer	1977	Popliteal cysts
Lukes et al	1980	
Simpson et al	1980	
Gompels and Darlington	1977	Rupture of popliteal cysts
Gebel et al	1978	
Desantos and Goldstein	1978	Delineation and origin of invasive osteogenic tumours
Kramps and Lenschow	1979	Bone cysts and bone tumours
Greenfield et al	1981	Disturbances of bone remodelling, and diseases of the skeletal system
Nassiri et al	1979	Behaviour of muscle tissue
Abendschein and Hyatt	1972	Consolidation of fractures
Hinkefuss	1974	
Gramlich et al	1978	
Leitgeb	*	Assessment of firmness of callus tissue
Stuhle et al	1980	Articular surface of patella
Porter et al	1978	Measurement of spinal canal in spinal stenosis
Stockdale and Finlay	1980	
Hawkes and Roberts	1980	
Kadziolka et al	1981	
Fornage et al	1984	Patellar tendon
Sattler and Harland	1988	Angiography of arthroses (?)
Sohn and Casser	1988	Menisci
Katthagen	1988	Review of sonography of the shoulder
Hedtmann and Fett	1988	Atlases and textbooks of ultrasound of the locomotor system
Graf and Schuler	1987	
Löffler	1989	

* Personal communication

logist K. Th. Dussig. The investigations of the cardiologists J. Edler and C. H. Hertz on the heart drew the attention of the professional world and led to the foundation of echocardiography. Nowadays it is not only possible to carry out fine needle punctures guided by ultrasound but it is also possible to use it intra-operatively.

Ultrasound in the locomotor system is a relatively recent development, because ultrasound beams are totally reflected by cortical bone. It began in 1974 when Kratochwil and Zweimüller showed the borders of invasively growing bone tumours against their surroundings. Kramps and Lenschow carried out examinations of the hip in adults with ultrasound as early as 1978. Structures in the bone itself could not be demonstrated because of the lack of penetration of the ultrasound wave through the bone. However, demonstration of the anatomy of the infant hip is much easier because the proximal end of the femur and the acetabulum are still unossified. Later, interest spread to hip sonography and from there to other parts of the locomotor system (Sattler and Harland 1988, Fornage et al. 1984). The historical development of ultrasound in the locomotor system is summarised in table 1.1.

1.1 Physical basis

1.1.1 Basic concepts

When considering the wave-like properties of ultrasound we usually borrow physical concepts from the world of optics. This analogy works because ultrasound spreads through the human body in a linear fashion similar to that of light when considered by wave optics. Also we occasionally meet – as in optics – the occurrence of the refraction and interference phenomena.

Sound propagates itself as longitudinal waves causing periodic variation of the density of the medium through which it passes. The frequency of these waves per second is given in hertz (Hz). The human ear can appreciate frequencies from 16 Hz to 20 kHz. Oscillations above the range of human hearing are known as *ultrasound*. The frequencies used for medical diagnosis lie between one and nine megahertz (MHz); for special areas 12 MHz may also be used.

The speed of sound in air is 300 metres per second (m/s). In acoustically dense material it rises. Thus in water it reaches 1500 m/s, in iron 6000 m/s. In bone the speed of conduction of sound varies between 2700 m/s and 4100 m/s (Nyborg 1977).

The ultrasound waves generally used diagnostically in human soft tissue are longitudinal waves with an average almost constant velocity of 1540 m/s. The frequencies used (1–12 MHz) produce wavelengths of 1.5 mm down to 0.128 mm.

Acoustic impulse sent out into the body is reflected at the surfaces or borders between tissues whose acoustic properties differ. The intensity of the reflection is dependent on the grade of the acoustic difference in the tissues and upon the angle of incidence of the ultrasound beam. The two most important acoustic properties of tissues are *density* and *elasticity*. From these arise the speed of the sound and the resistance to sound within the tissue: the so-called *acoustic impedance*. At interfaces between tissues with the same impedance value there is no reflection of sound. If there is a high difference between the impedances (as for example between connective tissues and air, or musculature and bone) almost the whole energy of the sound beam is reflected. Since, with the exception of air and bone, the acoustic impedance of various body tissues lie close together, the proportion of the energy reflected from an ultrasound beam is less than 1% of the impulse.

1.1.2 The production of ultrasound waves

In certain quartz crystals, mechanical deformation produces an electrical tension across the surface proportional to the degree of deformity. The reverse phenomenon can also be seen, in which an electrical tension placed across the crystal from outside can cause a change in the dimension of the crystals and an oscillation of the crystal can be produced. This is the so-called *piezo-electric effect*.

The nucleus of every ultrasound machine is thus an ultrasound transducer with its piezo-electric crystal. This probe head has two functions: first it serves as a transmitter with an intensity of 5–50 mW cm^{-2}, and it is also a receiver which can register intensities of 10^{-10} W cm^{-2}.

When ultrasound waves are transmitted from the transducer, these first run parallel and then begin to diverge like the waves of a beam of light. Thus, two areas develop within the ultrasound beam:

1. The *near field* in which the ultrasound waves are running parallel or may even be converging, and

2. The *far field* in which they diverge (Fig. 1.1).

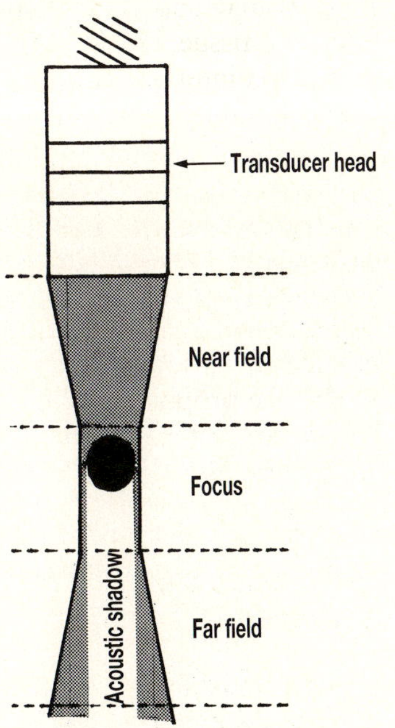

Fig. 1.1. Transducer with near and far fields, and an object in the focal zone

Between the near and the far fields is found the *focal zone* in which the resolution of the system is at its greatest. The resolution is defined as the smallest difference of two points on the image that can still be distinguished from each other on the sonogram.

For the sake of completeness we also need to distinguish between axial resolution (that is resolution in the direction of the ultrasound beam) and lateral resolution (resolution in the plane perpendicular to the ultrasound beam). Further technical and physical details can be found in the book by A. J. Goetz (1983).

Various other phenomena occur analogously to wave optics:

1.1.3 Refraction

Ultrasound waves passing from one medium to another can be refracted by the differing densities of the two media. Perpendicular incidence of the ultrasound beam is the only occasion when this refraction is not to be expected.

In homogeneous tissues the ultrasound waves propagate themselves in straight lines.

1.1.4 Diffraction

When the ultrasound meets an obstacle the ultrasound waves are diffracted (bent) around the obstruction. This diffraction phenomenon is dependent upon the frequency and becomes less noticeable with a rising frequency and shorter wavelength.

1.1.5 Scatter

The ultrasound wave only hits a border surface perpendicularly in the rarest of cases and there are no smooth interfaces in biological tissues. This means that there is usually marked scatter of the ultrasound waves. With rising frequency the strength of the scatter increases.

1.1.6 Absorption of ultrasound

An ultrasound wave passing through the body experiences a so-called "optical attenuation," principally through absorption and scatter. For this reason sound reflection is weaker from the deeper layers of tissue. A depth compensation control (or *depth gain control*) on the apparatus compensates for the weak echoes from the depths of the body.

An important practical point arises from these physical principles: a lower frequency gives a good depth of penetration but poor resolution, whereas a high frequency gives a lesser depth of penetration of the ultrasound but better resolution. A compromise has to be struck between these two extremes when choosing an ultrasound frequency, according to the organ being examined.

1.1.7 Methods of image production

The ultrasound beam has to be made to sweep from side to side so that the two dimensions of a 'slice' of tissue, or tomographic image, are covered by it. In principle, this can be done by three methods:

1. *Compound* scanning: a single probe is passed over the subject by hand: it has nowadays largely fallen out of use.

2. *Sector* scanning: the ultrasound head is made mechanically to rock or rotate. Ultrasound waves are passed out through a small window in the head of the probe to form an image the shape of the sector of a circle.

3. *Linear array* scanning: parallel ultrasound waves are sent out by a row (or array) of very small independent transducer crystals firing consecutively. The angle of insonation of the various parts of the picture remains uniform. A largely artefact-free demonstration of various tissues can be attained.

The so-called *curved array* attempts to combine the advantages of the sector and linear scans by a transducer of a compromise, curved shape.

1.1.8 Artefacts

Knowledge of certain imaging artefacts is important for the correct interpretation of a sonogram. For practical purposes in the hip joint the most important artefacts are:

(a) *Reverberation echoes*. These arise because of repeated reflection to and fro between two strongly reflecting surfaces. This causes lines of reflections lying parallel to and behind each other, which do not correspond to real surface borders. This phenomenon can be seen particularly with water standoff paths: the ultrasound beam zig-zags between the crystal of the ultrasound probe and the rubber membrane in which the water bath is contained.

(b) *Acoustic shadows*. These form behind surfaces at which the ultrasound beam is totally reflected, for example against the surface of bones, and appear as dark streaks behind the surface into which no sound can penetrate. In sonography of the hip, an ultrasound shadow causes the so-called half-moon phenomenon behind large femoral capital epiphyses. However acoustic shadows may also be important with well developed bony acetabular promontories when measurement points have to be determined.

Acoustic enhancement (reverse shadowing), the converse phenomenon to acoustic shadowing and seen behind structures which propagate the ultrasound wave very strongly, and electronic *amplifier noise* produced when imaging deep-lying structures, are of no significance in ultrasound of the infant hip.

1.2 Biological effects and questions of safety

The question of negative biological effects and the possibility of harming biological tissues continues to be brought up. Effects of ultrasound at very high intensities include: the development of heat (Rott, 1984), microstreaming, biological effects (Wood and Loomis, 1927), and chemical effects, leading to mutagenicity and teratogenicity (Abdulla et al 1971, Vegner et al. 1980). None of these has been found to produce an effect at diagnostic intensities[1].

Key Points

- Diagnostic ultrasound machines use wavelengths in the range of 1–12 MHz.

- Ultrasound transducers contain a piezo-electric crystal which both produces pulses of ultrasound and detects echoes from the tissues examined.

- Echoes are formed where the ultrasound beam meets an interface between two tissues of different acoustic impedance.

- Ultrasound beams have a near zone and a far zone separated by a focal zone where the resolution of the image is at its greatest.

- The ultrasound beam may also be refracted, diffracted, scattered or absorbed as it passes through the tissues. Some compensation for these is provided by the depth gain control.

- The best type of transducer for the examination of the hip is the linear array type.

- Artefacts seen in ultrasound images include reverberation echoes (seen against dense interfaces) and acoustic shadows (seen behind dense interfaces).

- Diagnostic ultrasound is completely safe.

---

[1] The Declaration of Biological Effects of Ultrasound in Mammals in vivo: American Institute for Ultrasound in Medicine, 1992

2 Ultrasound equipment

2.1 Superiority of real-time linear array transducers

Over the last few years, the older compound scanners have been replaced by real-time sector or linear scanners. These have much higher resolution and their 'real-time' or cinematic capability is invaluable in observing movement, particularly in the so-called stress or dynamic examinations. Beyond this, the choice of the best type of scan head (transducer) depends critically upon the type of examination being performed: for example, satisfactory examination of the menisci of the knee can only be done with a sector scanner, but the decision is less critical for examination of the shoulder.

In the case of the infant hip, the most basic observations – whether or not a femoral head is subluxed at all – have been made over the years with a variety of types of transducer. It was only when there came a demand for increasing precision, quantification and morphometric results in the hip joint that characteristic differences between the two types of scan-head became obvious. We formalised these observations by carrying out measurements of the speed of sound in the infant hip joint intra-operatively in vivo (Graf 1988). These supported the recommendation for linear transducers. Snelius' law of diffraction shows that misregistration of the angles between tissue planes due to refraction and diffraction of the ultrasound beams is minimised if the beams travel as nearly as possible parallel to each other as they pass through tissue. If the pulses of ultrasound are not parallel, then varying speeds of sound in the musculature and

in the hyaline femoral head, and oblique angles of incidence, allow variations in the refractive indices in the tissues to become apparent. These can be a cause of distortion of the image, leading to apparent increase in the angles at which surfaces and interfaces within the body lie relative to each other.

Independently of these methodical demands, the elongated shape of the linear transducer makes the procedure and handling of the infant during examination considerably easier. By this means, a strictly standardised procedure can be taught and learnt so that the production of a good hip sonogram does not depend completely upon the dexterity of the examiner.

2.2 Relative merits of linear and sector scanners

by Karl Schneider

2.2.1 Preliminary remarks

In Table 2.1 the characteristics of the three types of probe are reviewed as they apply to the examination and production of the images of the hip joint of infants. These advantages and disadvantages in imaging are valid in a similar fashion for the sonography of other joints.

Independent of the type of probe to be used, a probe with a frequency of at least 7.5 MHz should be used in neonates and in dystrophic infants up to the end of the third month because of its high resolution and because of the smaller near field. For all other patients a 5 MHz transducer is adequate.

Table 2.1. Comparison of the characteristics of ultrasound transducers as they affect their suitability for examination of the infant hip

	LINEAR	SECTOR	CONVEX
Attainment of the standard plane	Easy	More difficult	Easy
Contact between the femoral head and the skin	Contact without difficulty	Compression of the subcutaneous tissues	As for sector scanner
Effective size of image	Corresponds to the length of the transducer head	Smaller than 90° because of peripheral zone artefacts and 'zoom' phenomenon	Smaller than with a linear probe, compromised near zone
Near field	ca. 0.5 cm	With 5 MHz probe 1.5–2.5 cm; with 7.5 MHz probe 0.5–1.5 cm	1.5–2.5 cm
Resolution	Very good	Axial resolution good, lateral resolution poorer	Good
Artefacts	Rare, usually insignificant	Frequent, with misregistration and reverberations	Rare, usually insignificant

2.2.2 Finding the standard plane of section

Ultrasound of the infant hip depends upon finding exactly the standard plane of section, and it is easier to do this with a linear array transducer simply because of its physical shape: it has an obvious long axis, and this can be directly observed and correlated with the findings on the image as the probe lies against the patient's skin, much more easily than can be done with the rounded head of a sector scanner.

Tipping of the probe up and down, along the plane of section, is possible with both the sector and the convex type of probe. These errors of adjustment of sector and convex probes are of significance, as artefacts can arise from them (see table 2.1). Such possibilities for error are largely absent from linear transducers.

2.2.3 Contact of the ultrasound probe

The characteristics of coupling of an ultrasound transducer (i.e., close physical contact through the contact gel with the surface of the patient) depend upon its geometrical form. Linear transducers with a length of about 6–8 cm have special advantages as complete contact is possible with them at almost all ages. In sector and convex probes the contact is limited to a surface area of 1–2 square centimetres. This inadequate contact causes peripheral zone artefacts and can also lead to the subcutaneous fat tissue under the centre of the probe being pressed away. This in turn causes a reduction of the distance between the probe and hip joint, which can cause the near zone to reach down as far as diagnostically important structures such as the acetabular labrum and the perichondrium with 5 MHz ultrasound transducers in very small babies (Fig. 2.1).

These disadvantages of imaging in the near field can be avoided by use of a standoff but these in turn cause serious technical difficulties in the imaging of the correct plane of section.

2.2.4 Effective size of the image

With linear arrays the size of the image corresponds to the length of the transducer in contact with the patient. If a sector scanner is used then a smaller area than the potential maximum field of 90–100° is available because of inadequate contact and the peripheral field artefacts that this elicits. With some instruments, turning on the zoom facility causes a further reduction in the sector down to half its original value, for example a sector of only 60° instead of 90° (Figs. 2.1 and 2.2). The relative lack of a near-field artefact (see below) with linear transducers also increases the effective image size (Figs. 2.3, 2.4).

2.2.5 The near field

The near field is that part of the image lying immediately under the transducer in which no clear image can be produced for physical reasons. Its extent depends upon three parameters: the frequency of ultrasound being used, the dimensions of the transducer head and the focal depth. This near zone is considerably smaller with a linear transducer than with a sector scanner. With linear probes with a frequency of 5.0 MHz and a short focal depth, the near field measures under 1 cm deep and can thus be ignored (Figs. 2.3, 2.4). With sector scanners, the near field measures about 1.0 to 1.5 cm at 7.5 MHz, and at 5.0 MHz it stretches for 2 to 2.5 cm (Fig. 2.1, 2.2) (Walter).

This difficulty with sector scanners can be compensated for to some extent by the use of higher frequency probes, but then the better discrimination in the near field has to be set against the reduced depth of penetration.

Thus, it is possible to use a 7.5 MHz probe in infants up to the age of six months, and this enables structures close to the probe to be imaged adequately (Fig. 2.5). However, the inferior edge of the iliac bone may not be seen because it lies below 4 cm or so, and

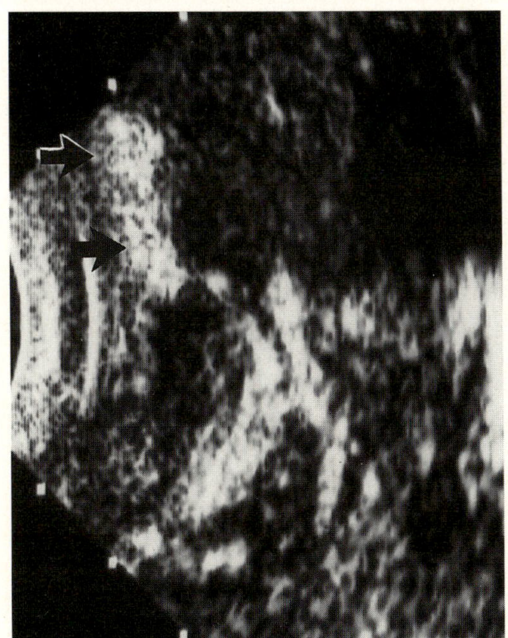

Fig. 2.1. Four week old baby. 5 MHz sector scanner. The iliac bone is shown as being grossly widened (arrow). The perichondrium and the acetabular labrum are drowned in reverberation echoes

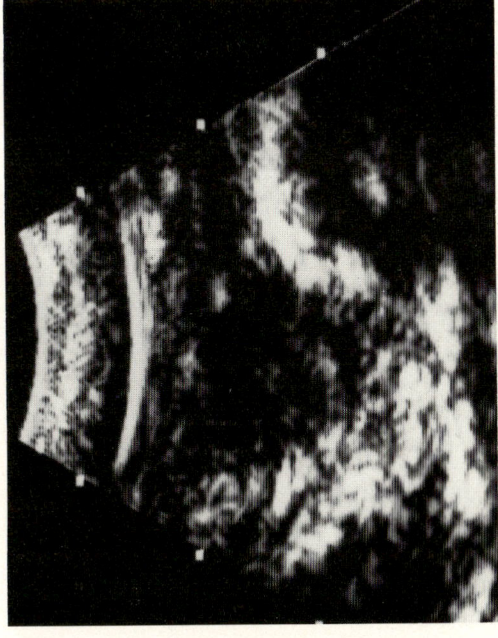

Fig. 2.2. The same patient as in figure 2.1; 5.0 MHz sector scanner, with the image maximally enlarged and reduction of the image sector to 60°. Angulation in the horizontal plane. The inferior border of the iliac bone is not demostrated

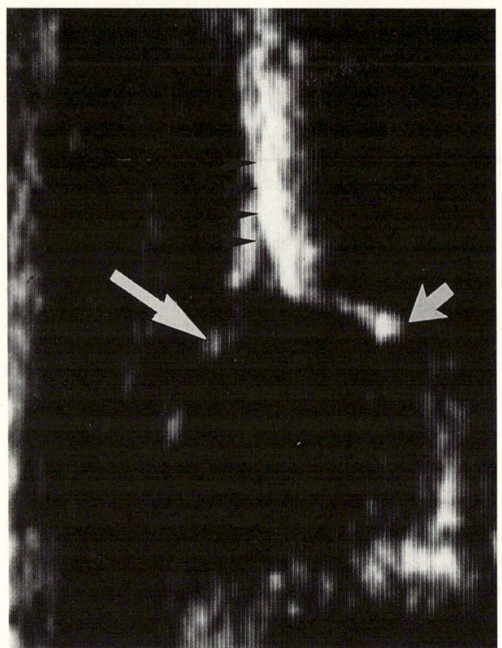

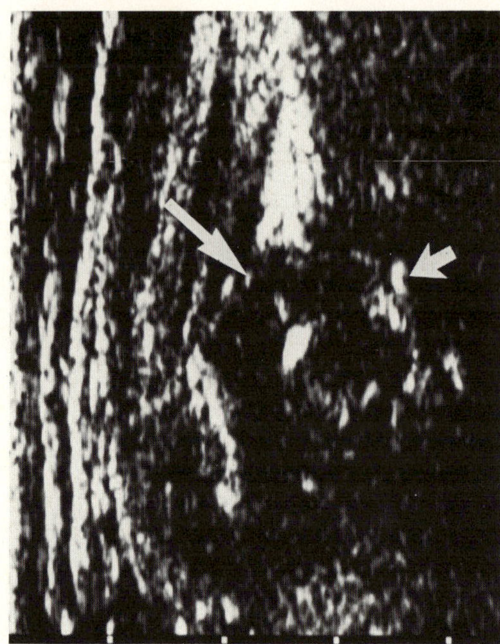

Fig. 2.3. The same patient as in figures 2.1 and 2.2; 5.0 MHZ linear transducer. All the relevant structures are demonstrated. Iliac bone (short arrow), acetabular labrum (long arrow). The junction between periosteum and perichondrium can be made out unambiguously (arrowheads)

Fig. 2.4. Five-month-old baby. The same patient as in figures 2.6 and 2.7; 6.0 MHz linear array transducer. Iliac bone (short arrow), acetabular labrum (long arrow) are adequately shown. The junction between periosteum and perichondrium is easily recognisable

is beyond the range of penetration of the probe. When a 5 MHz transducer is used the iliac tip can indeed be shown but structures in the near field are lost, such as the acetabular labrum, perichondrium and cartilaginous rim (Fig. 2.6). Convex transducers are not a great deal better (Fig. 2.7), and neither approach the capabilities of the linear transducer.

2.2.6 Artefacts

Artefacts dependent upon the ultrasound head are very rare with linear arrays and disturb the image only to a negligible extent. With mechanical sector scanners, artefacts are frequent (Fiegler, Winter). The main ones are reverberation echoes, which occur principally in the near zone (Fig. 2.1, 2.2), and two types of misregistration artefacts:

those that arise from tilting of the ultrasound probe in the horizontal plane (Graf) and those that are dependent upon maladjustment of the machine (Winter). Both types are of the utmost importance as they can lead to distortions in the representation of rounded or oval structures, for example the hip socket, and this in turn has an influence upon the measurement of angles. However, they can be avoided by carrying out regular quality controls with an ultrasound phantom (Winter).

The degree to which a curved array can minimise the disadvantages of a pure sector scanner and approach the specifications of a linear transducer can only be determined by further investigations.

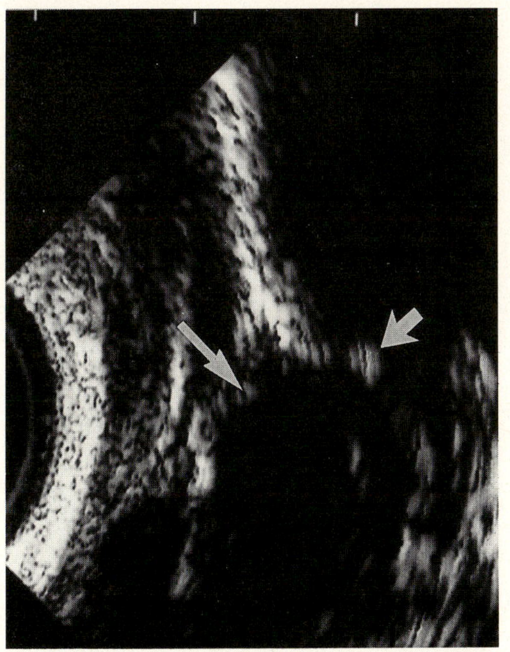

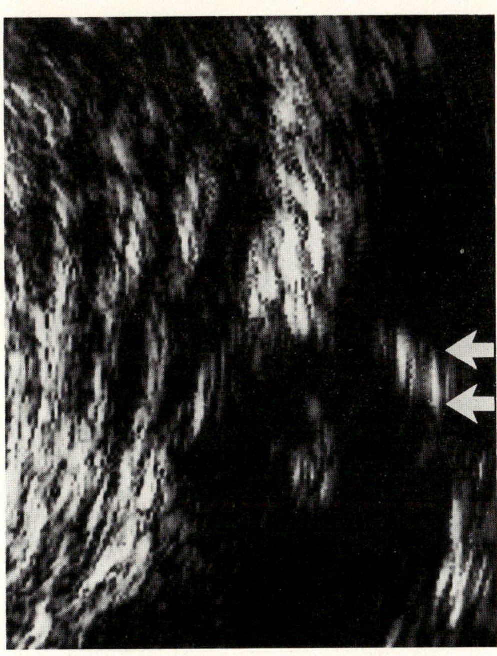

Fig. 2.5. Same patient as in figures 2.1–2.3; 7.5 MHz sector scanner. Iliac bone (short arrow), acetabular labrum (long arrow) are adequately demonstrated. The periosteal-perichondrial junction is not clearly recognisable

Fig. 2.6. The same patient as in figure 2.4. 5.0 MHz sector scanner. The lower edge of the iliac bone is somewhat widened (arrow), but is otherwise easily recognisable. The perichondrium, and acetabular labrum can only be dimly made out

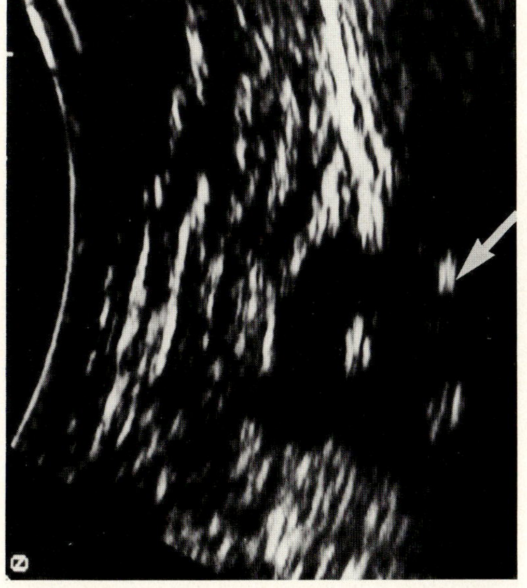

Fig. 2.7. The same patient as in figures 2.4 and 2.6; 5.0 MHz convex array transducer. The iliac bone is well shown (arrow). The acetabular labrum and the joint capsule are not adequately demonstrated. The junction between periosteum and perichondrium is not clearly recognisable

2.2.7 Literature

Fiegler, W. Artefakte in der Ultraschalldiagnostik. Fortschr. Röntgenstr. 138 (1983) 340–347
Graf, R., P. Schuler: Mögliche Winkelverzeichnungen am Säuglingshüftgelenk. In: R. Graf (Hrsg.): Sonographie am Stütz- und Bewegungsapparat bei Erwachsenen und Kindern. Edition Medizin VCH, Weinheim–Basel–Cambridge–New York 1988, 27–30
Walter, J. P.: Physics of high-resolution ultrasound – practical aspects. Rad. Clin. N. Amer. 23 (1985) 3–11
Winter, J., C. Kimme-Smith, W. King: Measurement accuracy of sonographic sector scanners. AJR 144 (1985) 645–648

2.3 Instrument settings

2.3.1 The acoustic output control

This determines the energy with which the tissue is insonated. Investigation of tissues lying deeper requires more acoustic energy.

2.3.2 The depth gain control

It is obvious that reflected echoes reduce in intensity with increasing depth, i.e., image-forming impulses from deep in the body are weaker. In order to produce an image of uniform brightness it is thus necessary to amplify those echoes coming from the depths of the patient more than the ones coming from the intermediate and superficial layers (Figs. 2.8a–c).

This control may also be known as the *timed gain control* because the echoes from the deeper structures are recognised by arriving back at the transducer later than those from the superficial ones, or as *swept gain* control or *depth compensation control.*

2.3.3 The contrast control

This works by filtering out weak echoes. Contours of organs can be demonstrated better in this way and their delineation against neighbouring organs can be considerably improved. In sonography of the infant hip a high contrast image is to be preferred with a 'hard' appearance. In contrast to this would be a softer picture with many grey scale steps as is practised in the abdomen or in sonography of the shoulder.

2.3.4 The focal depth

The depth of the focal zone can be adjusted on many modern ultrasound probes, thus affecting the relative sizes of the near and far fields as well. For examination of the infant hip a short focal depth should be selected, with the focus close to the transducer head.

2.3.5 Pre- and post-processing

The functions described above are set either before or during the acquisition of the image and are collectively referred to as *pre-processing.* The highest technology ultrasound machines with digital image processing can alter the image further in brightness and contrast once it is on the screen (*post-processing*).

Although the image can be made clearer for the viewer in some cases by altering these settings, no increase in the basic information can be obtained. This means that poor pre-processing can never be compensated for by post-processing however sophisticated and expensive it is.

The controls for the acoustic intensity, the depth gain and the contrast must be set so that the hyaline femoral head is echo-free or echo-poor (Fig. 2.8).

2.4 Choice of instrument

Technical requirements for ultrasound machines to be used for the infant hip have been laid down by the relevant professional association in Germany (the Federal Union of Insurance Fund Physicians) (Table 2.2). However some additional recommendations can be given:

Machines should have a facility for *attachment of 5 and 7.5 MHz transducers,* as it may be necessary to change quickly from one probe to another during the examination because of varying depths of penetration and resolving power.

Adequate pre- and post-processing can increase image quality considerably.

A *'freeze' button* on the transducer head or as a pedal are indispensable – a freeze button on the ultrasound machine itself alone is not adequate.

There should be an adequate *zoom* facility on the screen bearing in mind the minimum acceptable enlargement factor of 1 to 1.

The *facility to measure angles* for the quantification on the hip sonogram are useful but not necessary.

A *secondary video monitor* connected to the video output can be useful and brings the convenience that it can be positioned freely to face the examiner. Most accessory monitors produce an effective enlargement of the

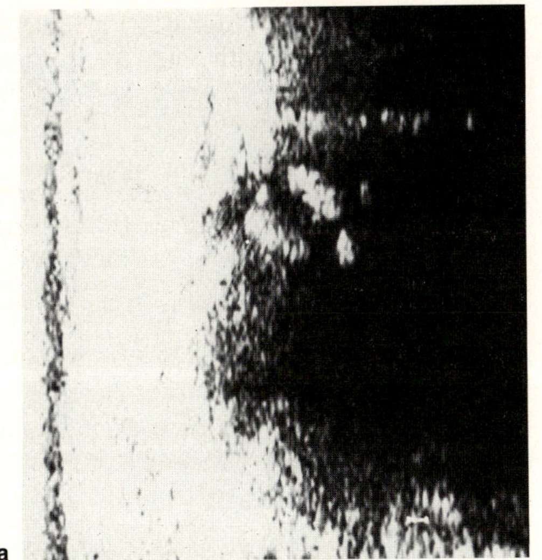

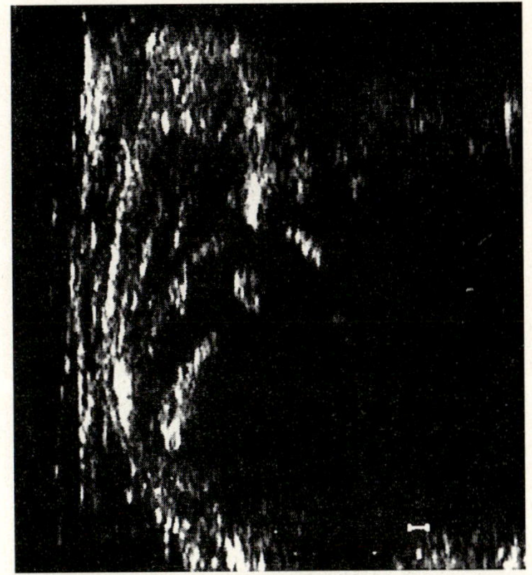

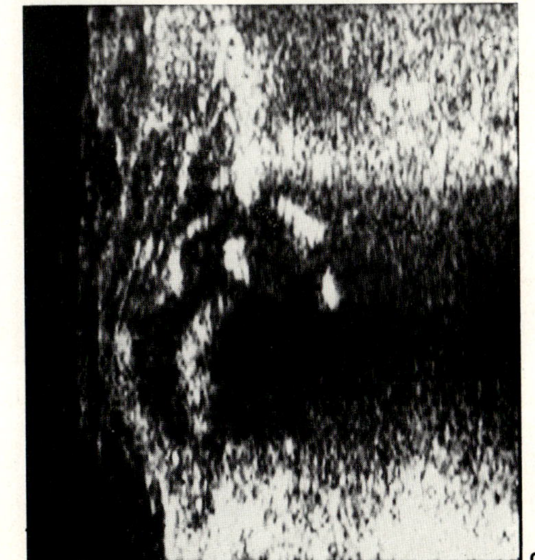

Fig. 2.8a–c. Depth gain control at various different settings. The direction of the transmitted ultrasound beam runs from left to right across the image (from the surface into the deeper layers).

a The initial attenuation has been turned up too high. The left-hand (superficial) half of he image is over-insonated.
b Correctly adjusted depth gain control with an evenly grey image from left to right.
c The right-hand half of the image is over-insonated. The echoes from the deeper structures are over-amplified.

image and this can facilitate diagnosis when the primary zoom controls are weak. The monitor can be tipped on its side to be brought into the usual projection for images of the hip, i.e. rotated to the right (see below).

2.5 Documentation of the hip sonogram

A suitable record should be made of each image taken, to allow a proper report to be made on it. The ruler giving the scale of the image should be retained.

2.5.1 Formal image criteria

Image magnification
As with the image on the screen, the hard copy should show the anatomy at no less than actual size, and preferably larger than this: this allows one to take measurements manually from the sonogram with precision.

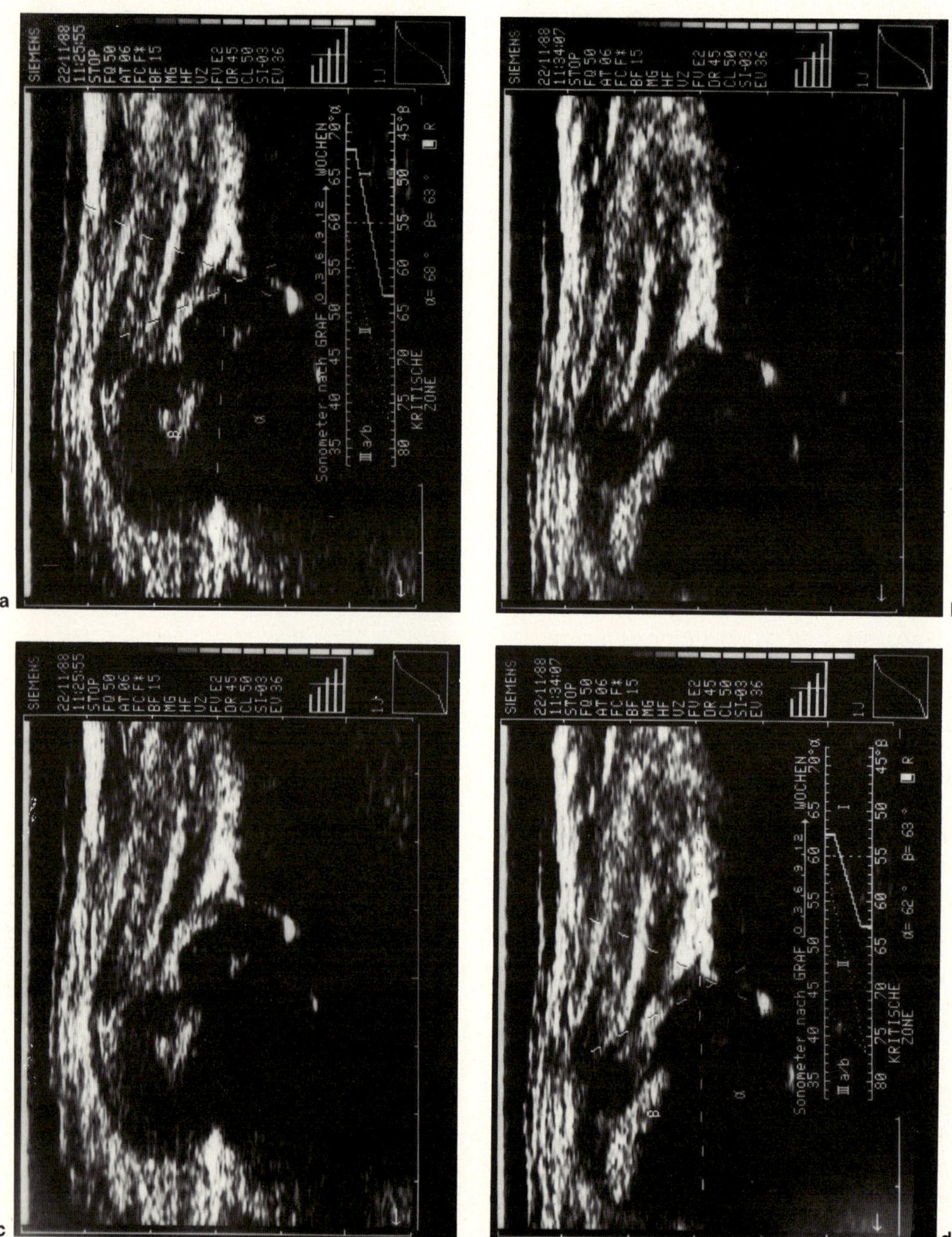

Fig. 2.9a–d. Example of hard-copy documentation with a multi-format camera, film size 18×24 cm. The correct method is to take two images of the standard section of each hip joint. The name and age should be given. One image of each is left free of measurement lines, to make sure that important details are not obscured. The other image has the measurement lines and the α and β angles drawn in, in this case electronically.

Table 2.2. Technical requirements for ultrasound machines used in sonography of the infant hip (German Federal Medical Association for Health Insurance Schemes). (Effective date 7 December 1985)

Two-dimensional image production	May be direct or with aid of an image storing device (analogue or digital)
Grey-scale (amplitude) steps	At least 16
Geometric distortion	Not more than ± 3% of the depth of the area being insonated. (Geometric inaccuracies of 1 mm are allowable.) These should be measured on a dedicated test object
Hard copy	Image documentation with scale information
Control of acoustic signal	Adjustable, calibrated output control and/or control of amplification of received signal; and depth gain control. Display of the selected values of signal processing
Transducer type	Ultrasound frequency 5 MHz, highest resolution (focal zone) in the depth range 0.5 cm to 5.0 cm.
Image enlargement	Image should be displayed on a scale of 1:1 or greater.

Projection of the image to the right

All hip sonograms, regardless of whether they come from a right or a left hip, should be projected so that they simulate an antero-posterior (AP) radiograph of a right hip. This practice has been retained because we have found from in-house audit that interpretation of the hip sonogram directly from the monitor leads to one-third fewer mistakes when the image is projected as right-sided than when it is projected as left-sided. The causes of the easier comprehension and interpretation of the right-sided 'standing' projection are neurophysiological in nature and have been discussed by Fischer (1985). The phenomenon is based upon the dominance of one side of the brain. A standard projection allows the examiner to become familiar with the anatomy, so that minimal changes in the relationships of the roofing of the acetabulum and the position of the femoral head are considerably more easily appreciated.

Documentation of two sonographic sections per joint

It is absolutely necessary to make two hard copy images of each hip examined. Both images are taken of the same standard plane, and small differences in the placing of the section through such structures as the acetabular roof can be compared between the two scans. This double-checking can frequently prevent misdiagnoses. If the angles are measured electronically on the screen, one image can be kept free of them so as not to obscure important details (Fig. 2.9).

2.6 Equipment for documentation

There are a great many types of equipment available commercially for the documentation of images and they vary a great deal in price. Look for a system which can produce an image of the dimensions of the original – many of them reduce the size of the image on the screen. Remember that the images must also be able to be archived conveniently, they must be immediately retrievable at follow up clinics, and the material of the hard copy must have a reasonable shelf life.

Key points

- Linear array transducers are the equipment of choice for ultrasound of the infant hip.

- They are easier to manipulate, and have a smaller near-field artefact than mechanical sector scanners.

- The parallel ultrasound beam they produce avoids misregistration of angles on the screen.

- They enable an image of at least actual size to be displayed.

- The main instrument settings to be considered are the controls for the acoustic output, depth gain, contrast, focal depth, and pre- and post-processing.

- Equipment is required with an adequate range of features.

- Some thought also needs to be given to the method for producing a permanent record of the examination (hard copy).

3 The infant hip: historical review of diagnostic modalities

3.1 Clinical diagnosis

The necessity for prompt initial *clinical examination* has always remained unchallenged, although the perceived value of the clinical examination has shown a basic shift in the age of hip sonography (see Chapter 13). Even before hip sonography became available, the safety of clinical diagnosis was thrown into doubt, dependent as it is upon many subjective factors (Ackermann 1984, Alby 1979, Von Rosen 1979, Weickert 1984). The so-called "silent cases" of hip dysplasia pose considerable difficulties in timely diagnosis (Breninek 1979, Tönnis 1987, Weil 1978).

3.2 Plain radiography

The interpretation of radiographs is difficult in the newborn period. They allow only a limited assessment because only the ossified parts of the hip joint can be considered (Heipertz and Maronna 1982) and this has led to some controversy (Tönnis 1984, Witt 1986, Werzinger 1989). It follows from this that radiographs are in general only indicated after the third to fourth month of life.

The A.P. view of the pelvis is beset with the following problems:

1. Radiation dose
2. Reduced sensitivity in the first three months of life
3. Errors of radiographic technique (rotation and tilting) and of positioning of the limbs can lead to poor results of measurements taken from the radiograph.

(Ultrasound of the hip remains reliable with the femur in a wide range of positions.)

3.3 Arthrography

Arthrography with its ability to show the non-ossified and soft parts of the hip joint cvomes very close to the capabilities of hip sonography. It is a good teaching method, allowing the operator to learn the anatomy so that the experience can be transferred to sonography (Fig. 3.1), and it has contributed a great deal to our understanding of the

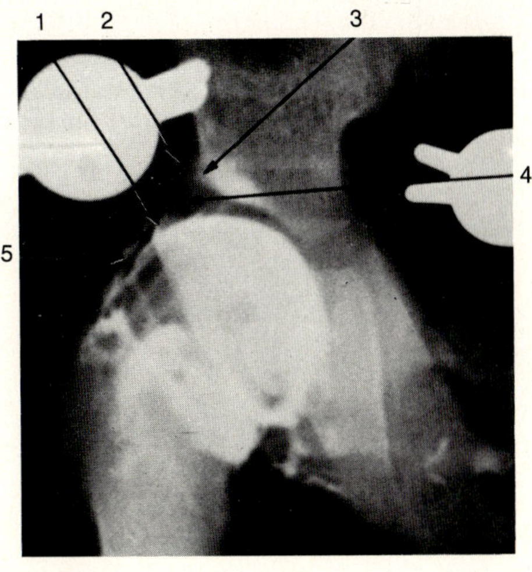

Fig. 3.1. Arthrography of the right hip (cadaver preparation).

1 Acetabular labrum
2 Perichondrium
3 Bony rim
4 Cartilaginous anlage of the acetabular roof (the 'cartilaginous rim')
5 Joint capsule

pathological mechanics of the process of subluxation (Faber 1938, Schwettlick 1976, Niethart and Gaertner 1982, Peic 1982, Buechelsberger 1982, Tönnis 1987). Drawbacks to arthrography such as invasiveness and radiation dose give sonography such an advantage over arthrography that its use is severely limited. Sonography can also recognise changes in patterns within the cartilage and this gives it a unique advantage.

3.4 Computed tomography and magnetic resonance imaging (MRI)

Cartilaginous parts of the acetabulum may also be appreciated with computed tomography (CT) and MRI. However, these methods require absolute freedom from motion artefact. Thus it is often necessary to sedate small children pharmacologically. Computed tomography of the infant hip joint is not a routine technique (Tönnis 1984) and should therefore only be used to answer specific questions and when other routine techniques have been exhausted. There is absolutely no question of it being used for hip subluxation or dysplasia of the hip in the form of screening (MRI also has these disadvantages although it produces outstanding images).

Key points

- Simplicity, ease of use, lack of invasiveness, and abilit of image the growth cartilage give ultrasound a unique advantage over plain radiography, arthrography, CT and MRI.

4 Development, anatomy and pathological anatomy

4.1 Development and anatomy

4.1.1 The femoral neck and head
(Fig. 4.1)

The hip consists largely of a cartilaginous precursor at birth. There is an ossification centre in the upper femoral epiphysis, and a second one spreads from a centre in the region of the greater trochanter. The epiphyseal centre for the femoral head appears between the second and eighth month of life, and that for the greater trochanter between the second and seventh year. However, the literature shows some variation in the reporting of the times of appearance of the femoral capital ossification centre: acceptable times of appearance vary from before the third or fourth month (Putti, 1929), through four months (Hilgenreiner, 1925) to over six months (Tönnis, 1984).

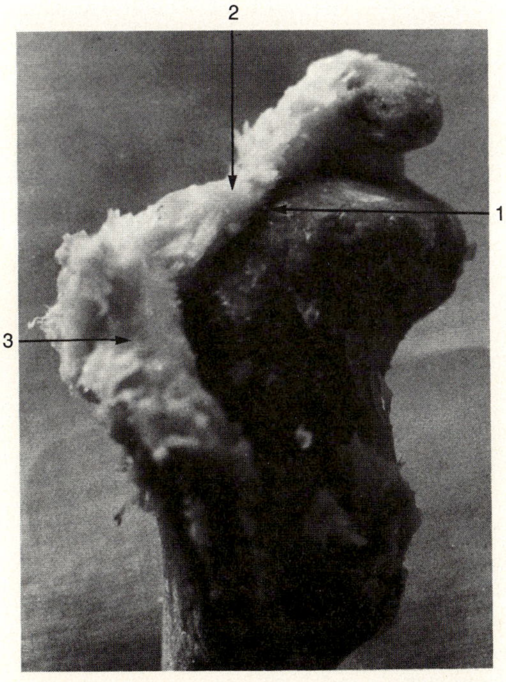

In fact, the presence of the femoral capital centre is of no consequence for ultrasound diagnosis in the hip (see below), but has some significance as a sign of maturity of the hip.

As long as there is no epiphyseal centre visible in the femoral head or greater trochanter, the border between the cartilaginous and bony parts is known as the *osteochondral junction* and corresponds to the edge of the primary diaphyseal ossification zone of the femur.

The shape of the semi-rounded osteochondral junction of the newborn period changes as the result of a varied growth potential, in that the medial parts of the growth plate grow considerably faster than the lateral parts. The initially shortened and compressed appearance of the femoral neck thus undergoes a stretching and increase in length. This age-dependent development of the osteochondral junction is sonographically significant, as it provides an important landmark for localisation of the femoral neck and head (Fig. 4.2).

Fig. 4.1. The proximal end of the femur with the ossification centre for the femoral head dissected free. The osteochondral junction (1) is exposed and the hyaline parts of the femoral neck (2) and the base of the trochanter (3) are clearly visible

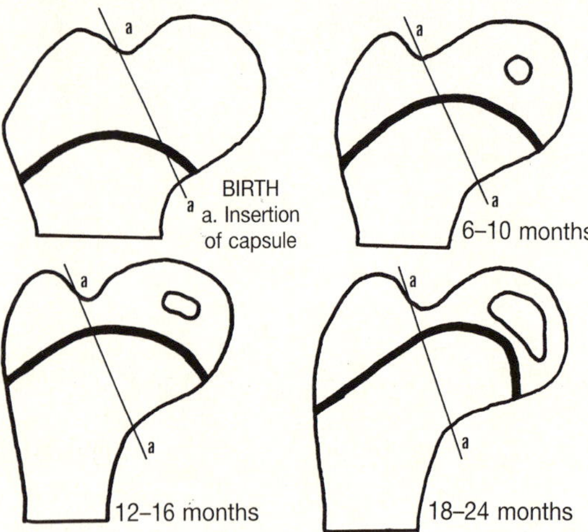

Fig. 4.2. The various directions of course of the cartilage bone junction depending upon age (after Batory 1982).

Birth [(a) insertion of capsule]
 6–10 months
12–16 months
18–24 months

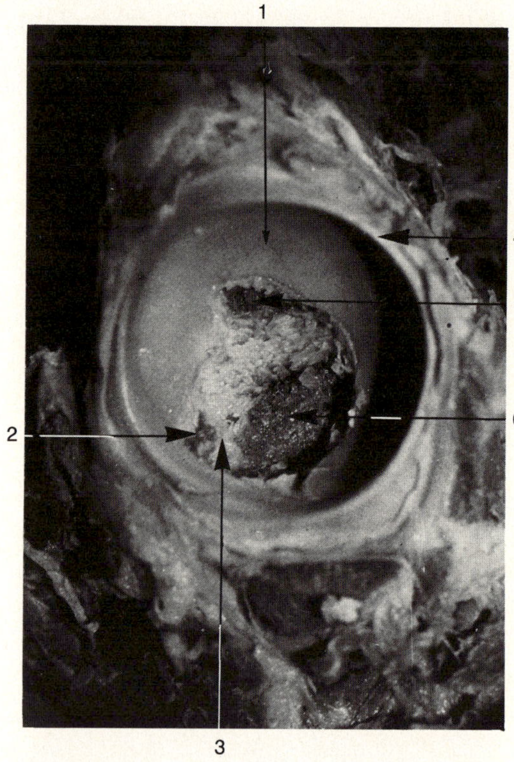

Fig. 4.3. View of a left acetabulum (dissection of a three month old infant). The ligament of the head of the femur and the tissues of the acetabular fossa have been removed to expose the base of the acetabulum.

1 Lunate fascia
2 Pubic bone
3 Descending arm of the triradiate cartilage
4 Acetabular labrum
5 Iliac bone
6 Ischial bone

4.1.2 The acetabulum (Fig. 4.3)

Recent investigations into the post-natal development of the hip joint come from the work of Dega (1973), Kopf (1970), Ponsetti (1978), Brueckl and Tönnis (1979), and Odgen (1983) to give only an incomplete review.

Three ossification centres for the iliac, ischial and pubic bones making up the *acetabulum* appear as early as the third and fourth month of fetal life (Fig. 4.3). Around these are formed the cartilaginous, not yet ossified parts. Otte (1970) gave a comprehensive description of the principles of growth of the pelvis. Harrison (1961) noted that the depth of the acetabulum is influenced decisively by the spherical femoral head. This also tallies with experience in untreated dislocation of the hip in older children: the depth and thus the total surface area of the acetabulum fail to develop further.

The fibrocartilaginous rim of the *acetabular labrum* encloses the acetabulum peripherally and its free edge passes over the region of the acetabular incisura (the transverse ligament). The bony, cartilaginous and accessory parts of the hip socket enclose more than half of the femoral head.

The *lunate surface* is a crescent-shaped gutter covered with articular cartilage which forms the articular surface over which the femoral head moves. The open mouth of the acetabular fossa faces downwards and forwards and in coronal section can be seen to consist of three layers:

The *deep layer* of the floor of the hip socket is formed medially of parts of the iliac, pubic and ischial bones connected by the horizontal and vertical arms of the triradiate cartilage. This cavity is covered with the *middle layer* consisting of loose fat and connective tissue. Lying on top of this, the *superficial layer* is formed of the ligament of the head of the femur running from the acetabular incisura into the femoral head.

4.2 Morbid anatomy

4.2.1 Morphology and morphological changes in the pelvis following dislocation

Anatomical and histological findings in cases of dislocation are described in order to give a better understanding of the sonographic images in disturbances of maturation of the hip. Detailed morphological investigations have been published by Bernbeck (1951), Oelkers (1961, 1981), Doer (1968) and Ponsetti (1978).

As already described, the head of the femur is more than half enclosed in the cartilaginous acetabulum and its labrum during early embryonic life (Fig. 4.4). If the primary formation of the hip socket is too shallow, it can lose its pivotal role in the development of the hip. Batory (1982) has demonstrated a shallow dysplastic socket as early as the fifth to sixth week of pregnancy in anatomical preparations. Oelkers (1981) prepared fetal pelves and succeeded in demonstrating a unilateral significant flattening of the hollow of the acetabulum with lateral displacement of the femoral head out of the pelvic ring. With the loss of the directive function of the socket, the femoral head is only held in by its capsule and this has only a tenuous fibrous binding to the acetabular labrum (Oelkers 1981, Ponsetti 1978).

One region important during the process of dislocation is the fibrocartilaginous acetabular labrum where it overlies the acetabular roof preformed in hyaline cartilage (Fig. 4.5) (Oelkers, 1961 to 1989). This point was referred to by Oelkers as the hypomochlion. This region is distinguished by forming a spring-like structural support for the labrum, strengthened by circular fibres with elastic elements. Thus the labrum is anchored against the hyaline roof of the socket by tissue of particularly tough construction.

During the process of dislocation itself, the femoral head glides in a craniodorsal direction over this hypomochlion as though over a firm wedge. As it does so, the fibrous elements of the acetabular labrum and the joint capsule are bent upwards at the back, while considerable parts of the acetabular roof consisting of hyaline growth cartilage remain in place (Fig. 4.6). Together, they form a broad trough-shaped seat for the dislocated femoral head (Figs. 4.6 to 4.11). This has a lip running round its inferior border, which is is crescent-shaped in three dimensions, running part of the way round the open mouth of the acetabulum, and forming the line of demarcation (the "neolimbus" of Ortolani) between the original acetabulum (the lunate surface) and the secondary acetabulum (the deformed acetabular labrum). This pad between the labrum and the bony pelvis is formed by the

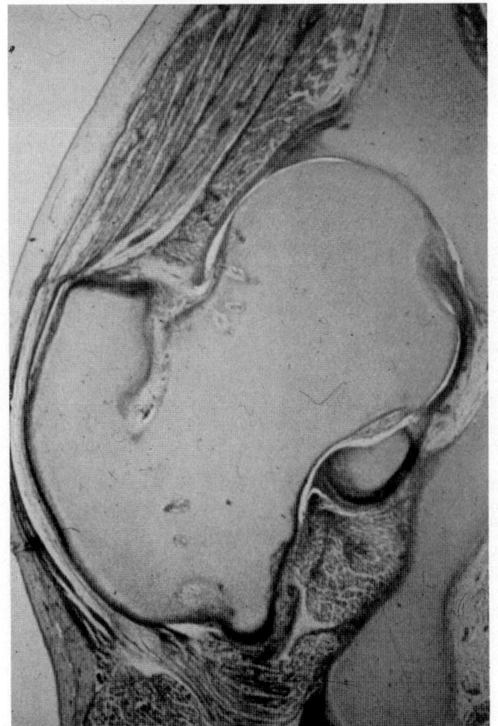

Fig. 4.4. Section through an embryonic hip joint

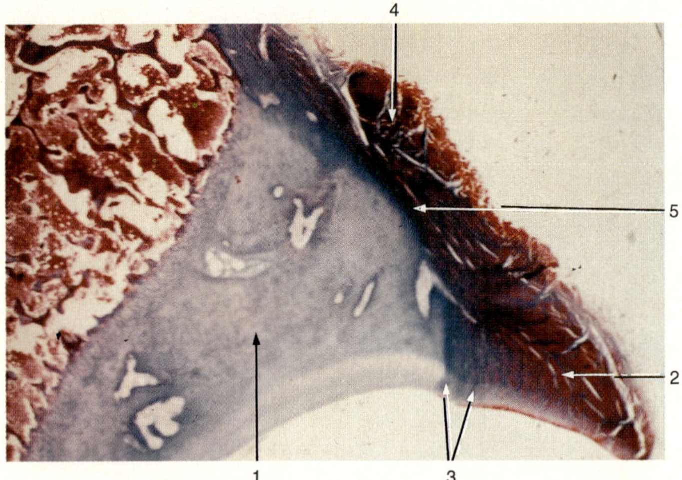

Fig. 4.5. Section through the cartilaginous part of the acetabular roof. Part of the acetabular roof preformed in hyaline cartilage (1) lies on the bony socket. The acetabular labrum (2) is particularly strongly fixed to the hypomochlion point (3) on the cartilaginous part of the acetabulum. (4) Joint capsule, (5) perichondrium

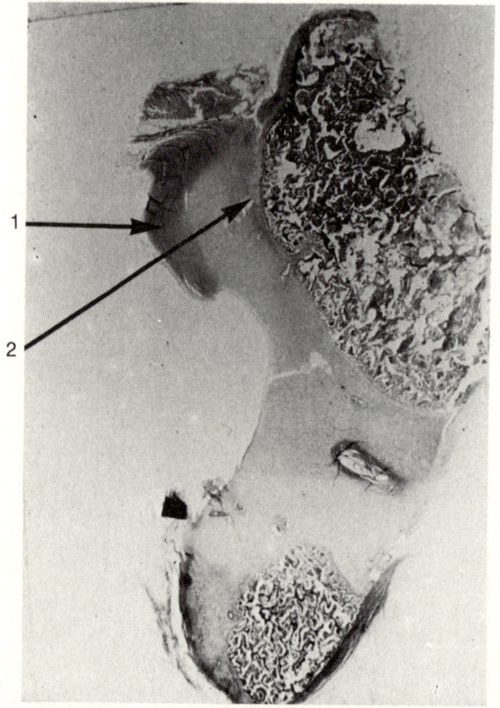

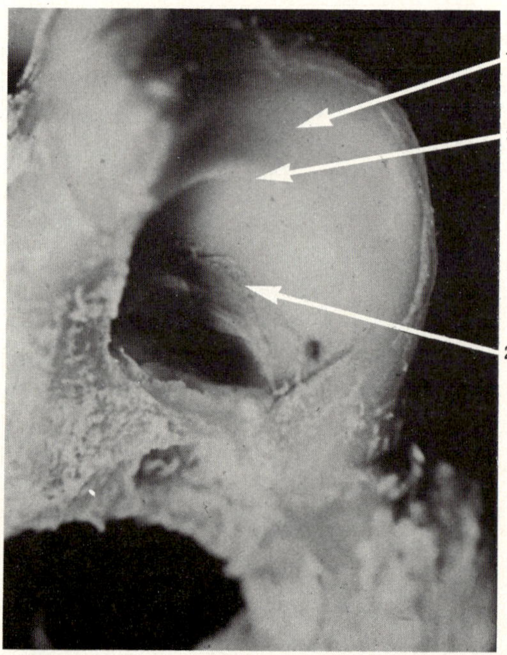

Fig. 4.6. Section of a right acetabulum, showing the acetabular labrum (1) dragged in a cranial direction with the joint capsule and the deformed cartilaginous acetabular roof. The regular columnar cartilage of the growth zone has undergone widespread destruction because of pressure and shearing forces (compare Fig. 4.12) (2)

Fig. 4.7. Left hip joint with dysplastic gutter (1) and original socket (2). (3) 'neolimbus' after Ortolani ('hypomochlion')

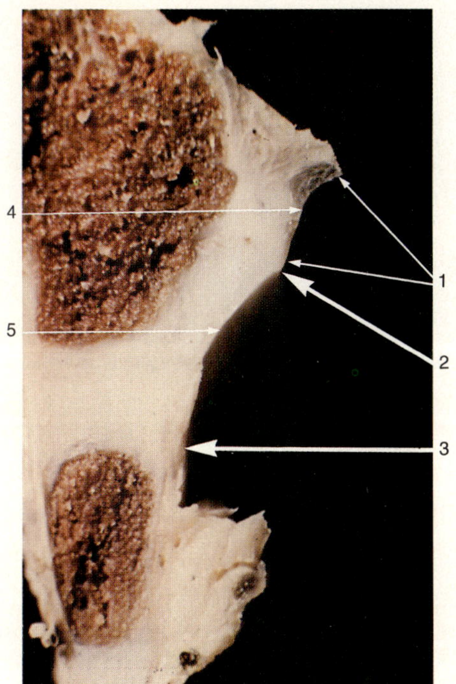

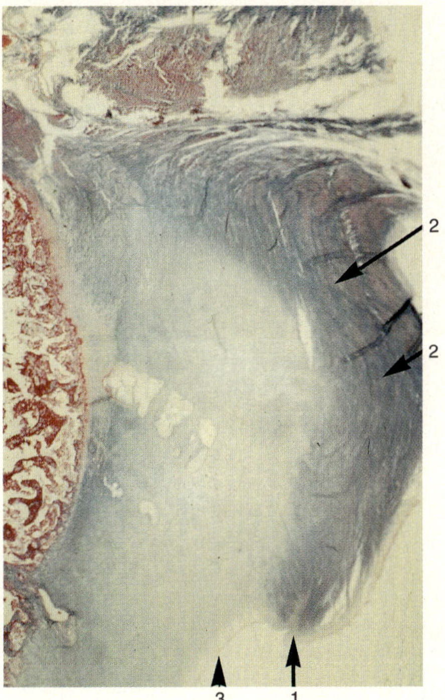

Fig. 4.8. Macroscopic section through a dysplastic socket. The labrum has been forced superiorly (1) and this and the hypomochlion point (2) are clearly visible. (3) acetabular fossa, (4) secondary socket (formed from the crushed labrum). (5) Lunate fascies (the original socket)

Fig. 4.9. Histological section corresponding to Fig. 4.8.

1 Hypomochlion point
2 The acetabular labrum deformed in a craniodorsal direction
3 Lunate fascia

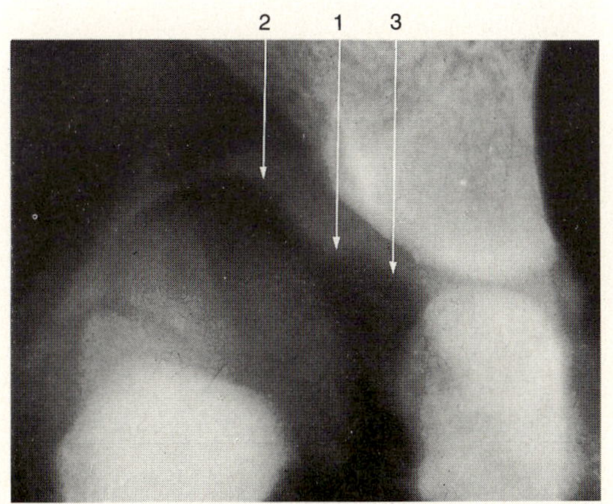

Fig. 4.10. Radiograph corresponding to the morbid anatomical situation in 4.8.

1 Hypomochlion
2 Apex of the acetabular labrum crushed cranially
3 Original socket (lunate fascia)

not yet ossified part of the cartilaginous roof of the acetabulum.

Thus the femoral head comes to lie in an immobile situation abutting the deformed acetabular labrum. The socket thus formed is open cranially, the so-called *dysplastic gutter* (Fig. 4.7).

4.2.2 Histological changes in the acetabulum in dislocation

Histology of the acetabular roof is distinguished by strictly regular architecture (Fig. 4.12). The growth zone is situated at the junction between the hyaline cartilaginous part of the acetabular roof and the bony socket. This shows a structure of columnar cartilage which is regular and typical for an epiphyseal junction. It is clear that when the hip joint

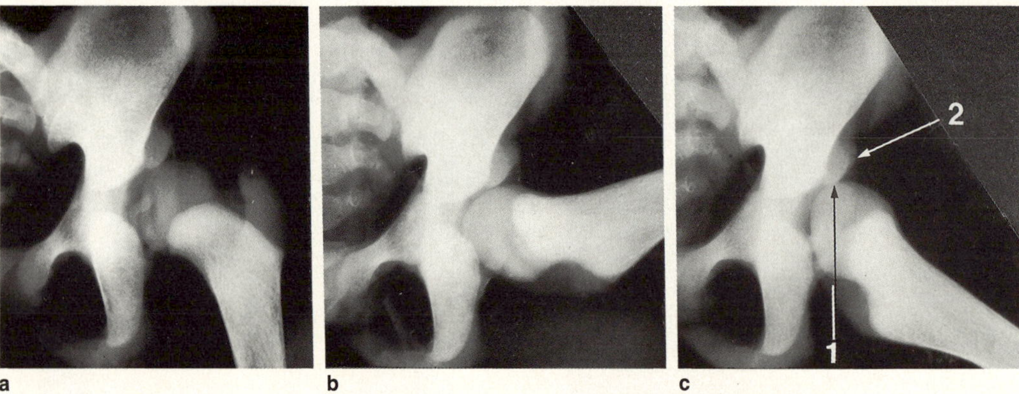

Fig. 4.11a–c. A relocated femoral head in various positions. The hypomochlion point (1) and the parts of the acetabular roof crushed upwards (the labrum, hyaline cartilage and joint cartilage) (2) are easily visible

becomes dislocated (Fig. 4.6), the forces of pressure, tension and shearing lead to a disturbance of this growth zone. It has also been experimentally demonstrated that application of pressure of various intensities and durations can lead to a limitation of the rate of growth (Rodegerts, Henning and Mathias, 1980). In adjacent areas not subject to high pressure, for example in the growth area of the triradiate cartilage, the histological structure remains almost normal (Fig. 4.13).

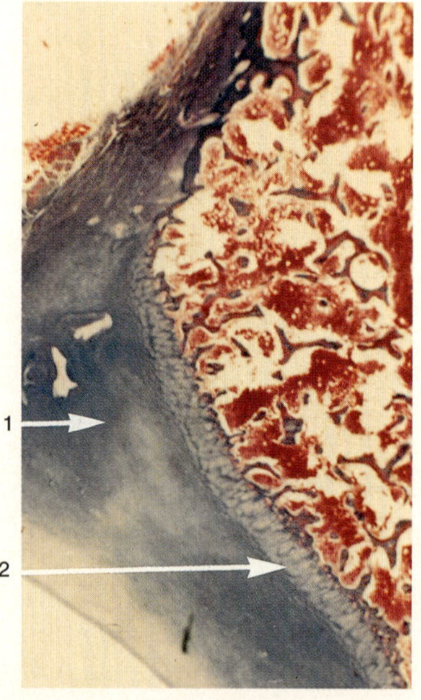

Fig. 4.12. Histology of a healthy acetabular roof area (coronal section). The cartilage of the hyaline acetabular roof (1) is separated by the growth zone of columnar cartilage (2) from the bony acetabular roof

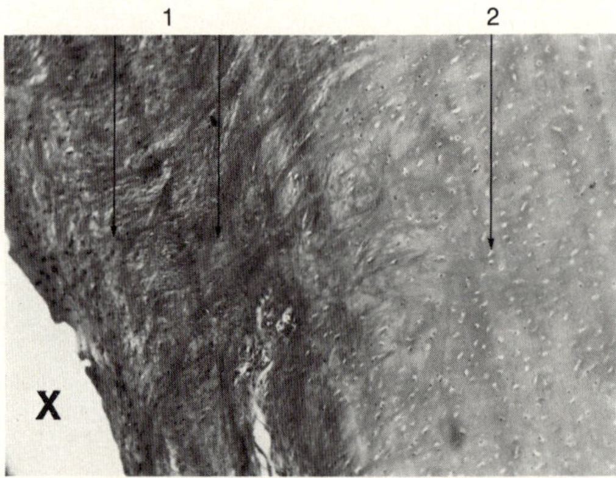

Fig. 4.13. Right acetabular roof cartilage in a subluxed hip. The transition zone has been highlighted by demasking of the collagenous fibres. The position of the dislocated femoral head is marked with an X. The cartilage of the acetabular roof outside of the zone of compression has not yet been markedly histologically changed.

1 Part of the cartilage with disturbed structure (zone of compression)

2 Histologically unremarkable cartilage

Furthermore, our own observations have shown that chondrocytes are transformed to fibrocytes under the influence of pressure and that the normal structure of the hyaline cartilage of the roof of the acetabulum is lost in regions of raised pressure. If these histological transformations and degenerative processes reach a certain stage they can, at least to some extent, be demonstrated sonographically. This growth arrest obviously has enormous therapeutic implications.

An inverted labrum composed of fibrocartilage can only be shown in the rare case of a dislocation which has occurred early in the fetal period from teratological causes (Ponsetti). Doer (1968) came to the same conclusion in his macroscopic examinations of the preparations of the dislocated hips in the collection of Ortolani.

I am grateful to Dr. Oelkers for providing me with Figs. 4.6 and 4.8 to 4.12. I am greatly indebted to Dr. Oelkers for his support over many years.

Key points

- Much of the skeleton of the hip is cartilaginous at birth.

- Ossification centres are found in the head of the femur, along the growth plate in the neck of the femur, and in the roof of the acetabulum.

- Normally the acetabulum and labrum enclose more than half of the femoral head.

- Contact between the femoral head and the acetabulum is necessary for the acetabulum to develop normally.

- During the process of dislocation, the femoral head glides craniodorsally and the soft tissues of the acetabular roof form a shallow 'false acetabulum' in which it lodges.

- Abnormal pressure by the femoral head on the acetabular roof causes fibrous degeneration of the hyaline cartilage and arrest of growth.

5 Sonographic morphology of the infant hip

5.1 The superficial soft tissues

Nowadays the appropriate method for diagnosing dysplasia and dislocation is the so-called 'coronal' slice, that is with the ultrasound beam directed in the coronal plane. This produces sonograms that are similar to an anatomical coronal cut through the hip joint (Figs. 5.1, 5.2). In Figure 5.3 the ultrasound beam penetrates from the lateral (left) s ide towards the medial (right) side. It traverses first the skin then the subcutaneous tissues, the fascia lata, the gluteal musculature and the septa lying between them. The intermuscular septa are more strongly echogenic than the intervening muscles.

Fig. 5.1. Coronal cut through a right hip joint (from A. Waldeyer: Anatomie des Menschen, part 1, 7th edition. De Gruyter, Berlin 1972)

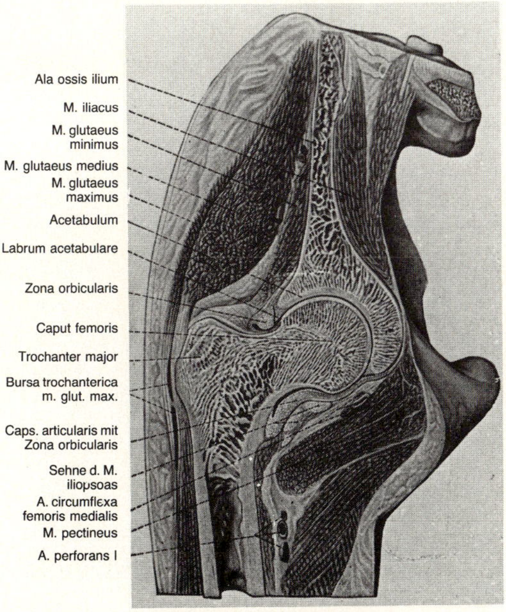

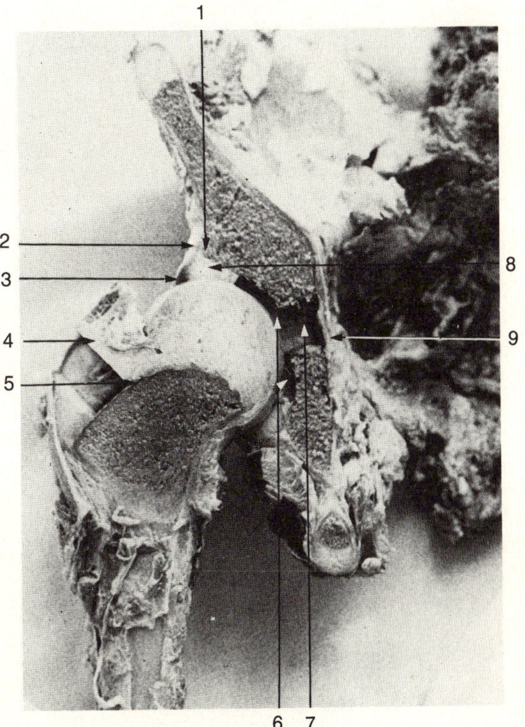

Fig. 5.2. Dissected section of a child's hip joint, corresponding to Figure 5.1.

1 Bony acetabular rim
2 Perichondrium and periosteum of the ileum
3 Acetabular labrum
4 Greater trochanter
5 Osteochondral junction ot the proximal end of the femur
6 Acetabular fossa dissected free
7 Triradiate cartilage dissected free
8 Acetabular roof preformed in cartilage
9 Periosteum on the inner wall of the pelvis

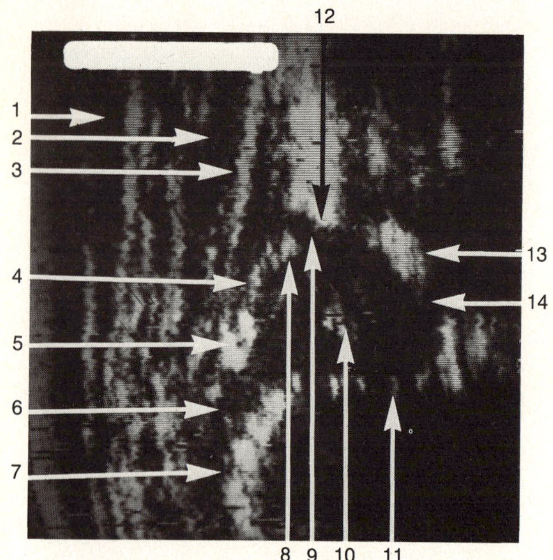

Fig. 5.3. Sonogram of a right hip.

 1 Subcutaneous fat
 2 Gluteal musculature
 3 Intermuscular septum
 4 Joint capsule
 5 Connective tissue folds of joint capsule and the perichondrium of the femoral neck
 6 Part of the femoral neck preformed in cartilage
 7 Osteochondral junction
 8 Acetabular labrum
 9 Acetabular rim preformed in cartilage
10 Femoral capital ossification centre
11 Acoustic palisade of the angulated osteochondral junction
12 Bony rim
13 Iliac bone
14 Triradiate cartilage

5.2 The proximal end of the femur

The proximal end of the femur is made of hyaline cartilage. Examination of these parts in a water-bath confirms that they form echo-poor areas, so-called 'echo gaps'. The proximal end of the femur consists of:

1. The *head of the femur*, possibly with a bony epiphyseal centre. (With well-adjusted ultrasound apparatus of high clarity it may be possible in certain cases to find small worm or threadlike reflexes in the hyaline part of the femoral head whose position can be seen to be fixed when the hip is rotated. These correspond to the echoes of vessels in the hyaline part of the femoral head that can also be seen in macroscopic sections (Fig. 5.4);

2. *The greater trochanter*. In contrast to the head of the femur, the upper surface of the greater trochanter is not smooth but is roughened by the tendons of the gluteal musculature radiating into it (Fig. 5.4), causing an irregular echo along its peripheral edge (Fig. 5.5);

3. The cup-shaped *cranial part of the neck* of the femur. This is bordered on the caudal side by the osteochondral junction and on its other sides by the joint capsule inserting on to the femoral neck. The femoral neck is short and the greater trochanter almost 'leans' against the femoral head (Fig. 5.6).

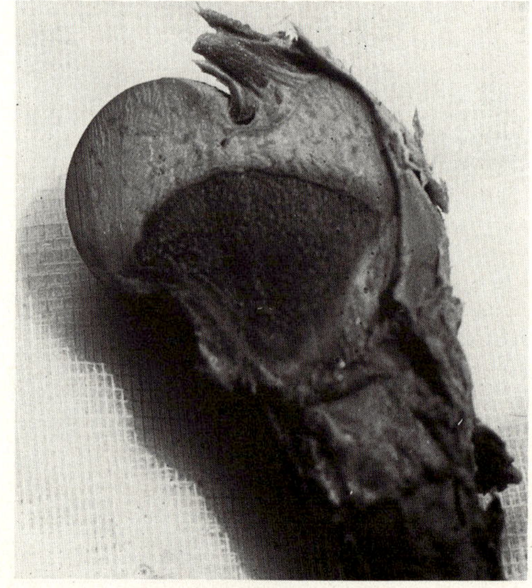

Fig. 5.4. Section through the proximal end of the femur. The bowed shape of the osteochondral junction and the greater trochanter with the ligamentous insertions are clearly visible. The truncated blood vessels and the hyaline cartilage are clearly to be seen

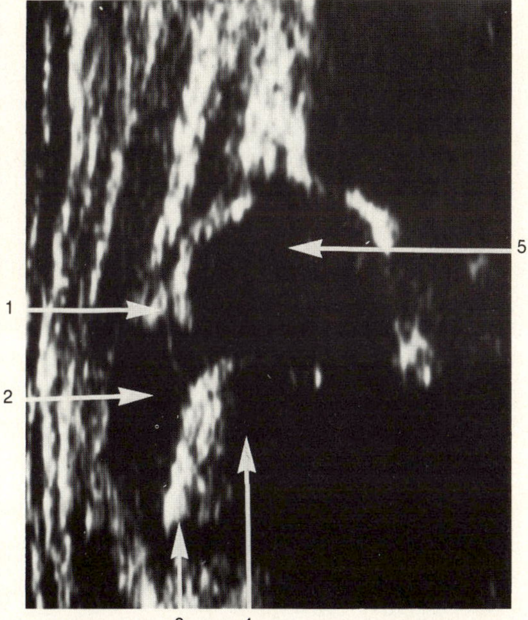

Fig. 5.5. Sonogram of the right hip. To distinguish between echo gaps and acoustic shadows

1 The connective tissue fold.
2 Echo gap of the base of the greater trochanter and the femoral neck preformed in cartilage
3 The osteochondral border
4 Acoustic shadow (bony part of the femoral neck)
5 Echo gap of the hyaline cartilaginous femoral head

5.2.1 The osteochondral junction

The osteochondral junction is a particularly important landmark in difficult cases for the identification of the femoral neck and head, and can considerably simplify interpretation for the examiner in grossly dislocated hips.

As no cartilaginous parts can be seen separately on radiographs, the cranial end of the femur as seen on a radiograph is formed by this osteochondral junction, which is bowed or formed like the head of a mushroom (Fig. 5.7). It causes total reflection of the ultrasound wave and shows as a strong echogenicity: this strong reflectivity is explained by the fact that the osteochondral junction is not a narrow sharply contoured border, but a wide and structurally inhomogeneous band. In Figure 5.6 the wide, curved, inhomogeneous zone of the osteochondral junction can be clearly seen. It divides the femoral neck into a peripheral part in hyaline cartilage, which forms a hood-like, echo-poor cap to the bony part lying underneath and medially.

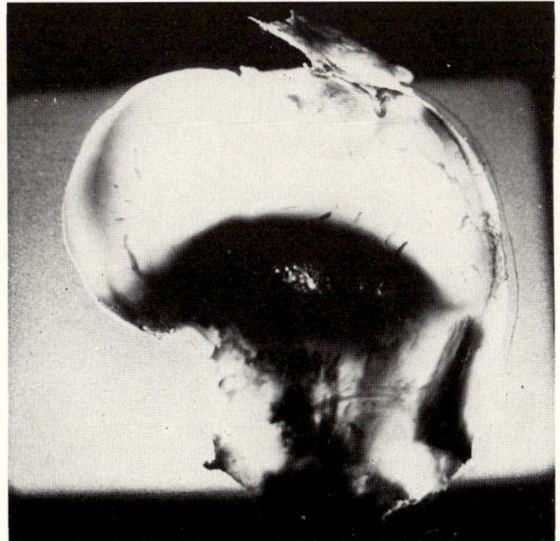

Fig. 5.6. Diaphanogram of the proximal end of the femur. The bowed course of the osteochondral junction can clearly be seen to be unsharp because of its inhomogeneity

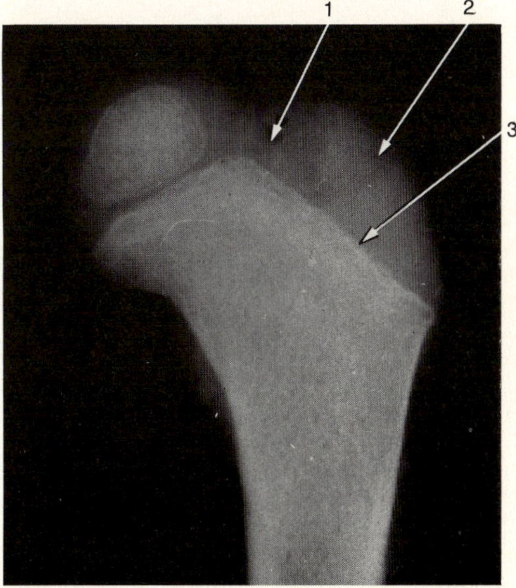

Fig. 5.7. Radiograph of the proximal end of the femur.

1 The femoral neck preformed in hyaline cartilage with the connective tissue fold.
2 Greater trochanter
3 The sloping osteochondral junction

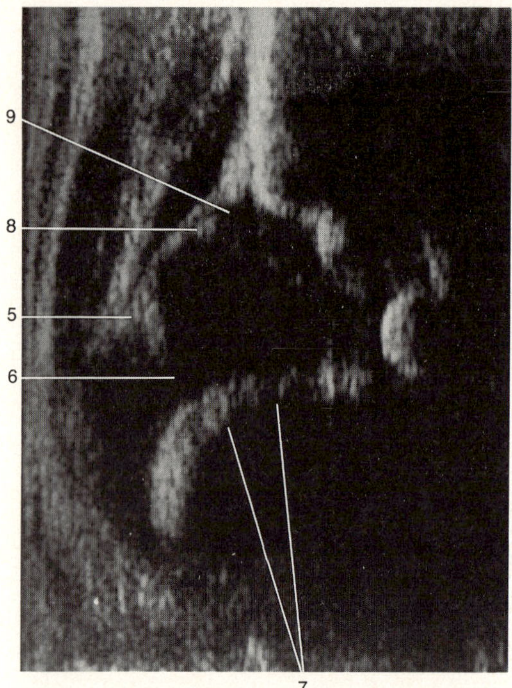

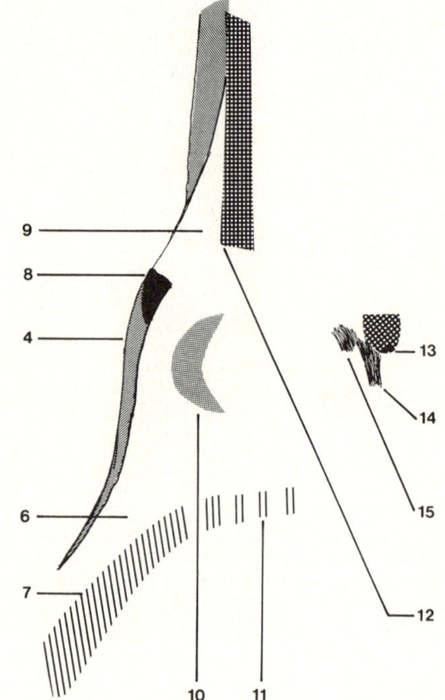

Fig. 5.8. Neonatal hip with a rounded osteochondral junction (7) which is demonstrable right into the depth of the acetabulum. Key as in Figure 5.3

Fig. 5.9. Schematic drawing of a right hip corresponding to Figs. 5.3 and 5.8. With the ultrasound waves approaching from the lateral side, only the outer side of the large femoral capital ossification centre can be shown. The medial side passes into the acoustic shadow (half moon phenomenon). Key as in Figs. 5.3 and 5.8.

14 Tissues of the acetabular fossa
15 Central fovea of the femoral head

The shape of the osteochondral junction changes with the child's age because of the varying strengths of the growth potentials of the medial and lateral parts of the femoral neck:

a) In neonates the osteochondral junction still rises as a bow and can be followed right into the depth of the acetabulum (Figs. 5.6, 5.8).

b) As the infant grows, the osteochondral junction becomes more angulated at its medial end, and begins to project between the femoral head and neck (as in Fig. 5.7). Thus the medial limb of the osteochondral junction falls more and more into the acoustic shadow of the bony part of the femoral neck lying laterally and it can then often only be made out as a palisade of echogenic stripes running parallel to each other (the *acoustic palisade* – Figs. 5.3 and 5.9).

c) In yet older infants the medial and lateral arms of the osteochondral junction fold over even more so that the medial arm falls not only partly but completely into the acoustic shadow of the bony part of the femoral neck lying before it (Figs. 5.7, 5.10). In these cases the medial part of the osteochondral junction cannot be demonstrated any more at all. Naturally this phenomenon of the demonstrability of the medial part of the osteochondral junction depends upon the positioning, and one can see more or less of it by abducting or adducting the hip.

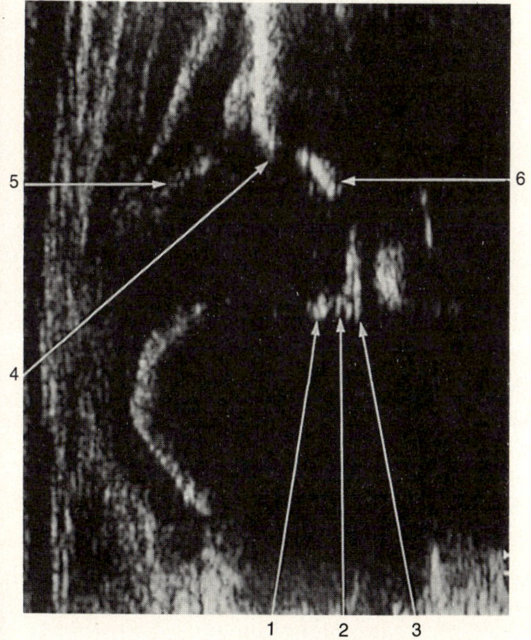

Fig. 5.10. Three layers of echogenicity in the base of the acetabulum (three month old joint).

1 Ligament of the head of the femur
2 Echo of the tissue of the acetabular fossa
3 Perichondrium of the triradiate cartilage
4 The bony acetabular rim
5 Joint capsule
6 Iliac bone

Note that there are two distinct areas at the end of the femur, each of which produces an echo-free zone by a different mechanism:

1. The *hyaline cartilaginous* parts which possess none or only very little intrinsic echogenicity (the '*echo gaps*'), and

2. the bony parts of the proximal end of the femur. These cause complete blockade of the ultrasound beam and thus form an echo-free *acoustic shadow* behind them (Fig. 5.5).

5.2.2 The connective tissue (capsular) fold

Just superficial to the hyaline head of the femur, the ultrasound beam first meets the echogenic collagenous joint capsule which borders the femoral head on its peripheral side. The joint capsule passes inferiorly, lying against the proximal part of the hyaline femoral neck, and at the junction with the greater trochanter it forms a fold of tissue (Fig. 5.3), commonly (if inaccurately) referred to as the *capsular fold*. Thus the perichondrium of the femoral neck and the greater trochanter come to lie closely applied to one another in this folded area. This gives rise to two parallel, strongly echogenic stripes of reflections lying close to each other, or sometimes to a conglomeration of echoes so that the folded area appears as a thick echogenic spot. Inexperienced operators or those with a lack of understanding of topography can mistake this echogenic zone of folded tissue for the acetabular labrum (compare Figures 5.3 and 5.8).

5.2.3 The femoral capital ossification centre

As the ultrasound beam passes through the hyaline femoral head it meets the ossification centre if one is present. The ossification centre certainly does not automatically lie in the middle of the femoral head.

The appearance of the femoral capital ossification centre can be seen on the sonogram 4–6 weeks earlier than in the plain radiograph. This is because the echo-poor or echo-free appearance of the femoral head is lost as soon as condensation of cells at an early stage of ossification gives rise to inhomogeneities of the histological and thus of the sonographic structure. The centre can be seen on the radiograph only when deposition of calcium salts has begun, at a considerably later stage of the overall process.

As children grow, so there is a tendency for enlargement of their femoral heads and increase in size of the ossification centres within them, and this can cause obscuration of the depths of the iliac fossa. This causes increasing difficulties with orientation of the ultrasound plane in the depths of the acetabulum as the inferior point of the ilium disappears into the acoustic shadow of the capital epiphysis, and forms a major limitation to hip sonography.

Morphologically, the femoral capital ossification centre is not always round, but may sometimes be oval or amoeboid in shape; also it does not always lie in the centre of the femoral head. If the acoustic plane meets a prominence of the femoral capital ossification centre then the resulting reflex may be small. On the other hand if it meets the widest diameter the reflex may be large. Since the position and contour of the femoral ossification centre is not known a priori, the plane of insonation does not in any way meet the ossification centre at a reproducible position. Thus an assessment of the size of the femoral ossification centre cannot be carried out in a reproducible fashion sonographically.

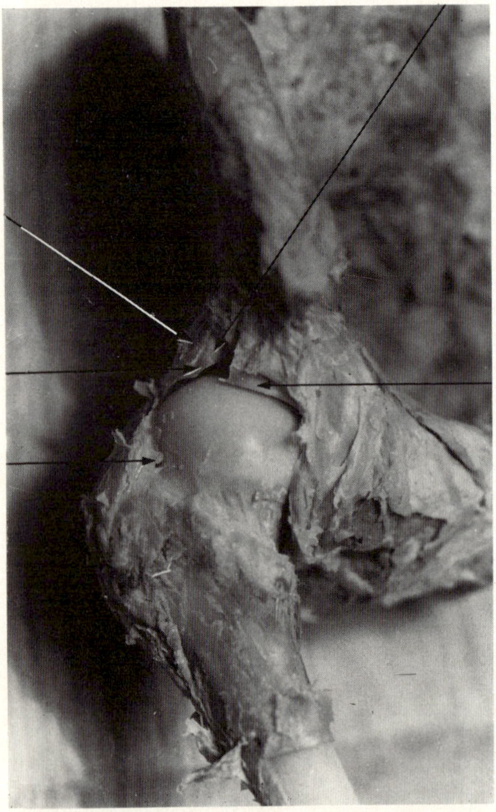

When the femoral capital epiphysis is very large only its lateral side can be demonstrated. Medial parts disappear into the acoustic shadow, giving the so-called *half-moon phenomenon* (Figs. 5.9, 5.14). Because of this half-moon phenomenon the femoral capital ossification centre may appear to be displaced laterally, and it cannot be used for diagnosis in the way that is done in plain radiography. For example, it is common practice on a radiograph to construct the Hilgenreiner line (a straight line passing through both triradiate cartilages), together with a perpendicular dropped from the acetabular rim, in order to show that the centre of the femoral head lies clearly inferomedial to the crossing-point of the lines. Even when this test is normal, the half-moon phenomenon (representing as it does only the lateral rim of the femoral head ossification centre) will often lie lateral to the vertical line. This may often lead beginners erroneously to report that the femoral ossification centre is laterally displaced because the hip is subluxed.

Fig. 5.11. Anatomical preparation of a right hip.
1 Perichondrium
2 Acetabular labrum
3 Connective tissue fold of joint capsule connected to the perichondrium of the femoral neck and the greater trochanter
4 Cartilaginous part of the acetabular roof
5 Free edge of the acetabular labrum jutting into the joint

5.3 The acetabular roof

5.3.1 The parts of the acetabular roof

The hyaline cartilage model of the acetabular roof has a central significance in hip sonography: all types of disturbances of maturation of the hip leave a mark here. Classification of hip abnormalities depends absolutely upon clear and unambiguous identification of its various parts.

The acetabular roof consists of cartilaginous and bony parts. The cartilaginous part is roughly triangular in shape and sits astride the femoral head, 'grasping' it. It is not equally large in every infant hip and is not uniformly easy to demonstrate sono-

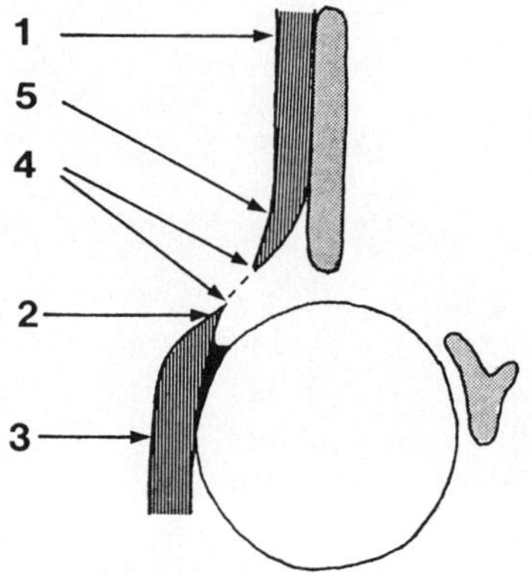

Fig. 5.12. The perichondrial gap. The strip of tissue of the periosteum (1), perichondrium (2) and joint capsule (3) is not equally wide throughout. The transition from joint capsule to perichondrium is abrupt while the transition from periosteum to perichondrium is gradual. Through the thin perichondrium can be seen the perichondrial gap (4).

5 Proximal perichondrium

graphically. It is bordered laterally by the periosteum and perichondrium, inferolaterally by the fibrocartilaginous acetabular labrum, and medially by the bony part, formed by the wall of the iliac bone (Fig. 5.15, 5.16).

5.3.2 The perichondrium

The superior part of the perichondrium, referred to as the 'proximal' part, is fairly thick and therefore strongly echogenic. Caudal to this, it undergoes a pronounced anatomical thinning. With standard adjustment of the ultrasound apparatus it may happen that this thin strip of perichondrium cannot be demonstrated and the lateral border of the lower part of the cartilaginous acetabular roof appears to be missing. This apparently missing border is referred to as the 'perichondrial gap' (Figs. 5.11–5.13).

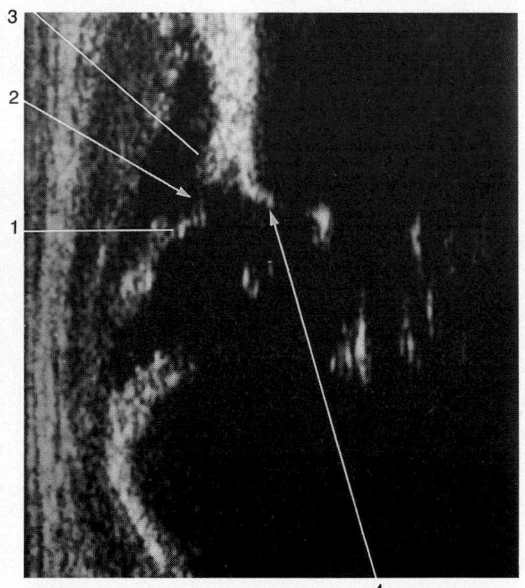

Fig. 5.13a. Sonogram with perichondrial gap.

1 Acetabular labrum
2 Perichondrial gap
3 Proximal perichondrium
4 Bony rim

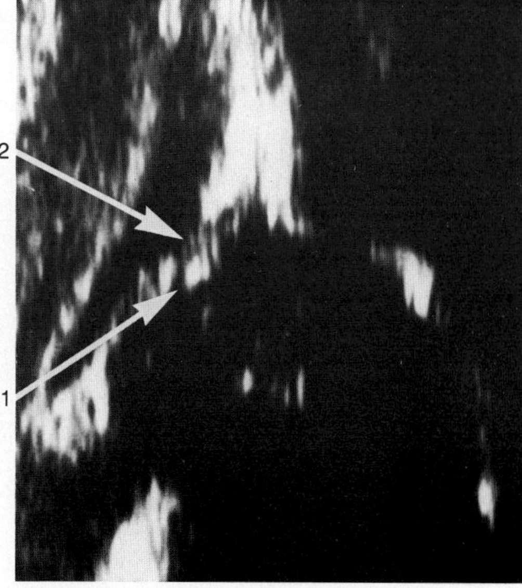

Fig. 5.13b. Here the perichondrial gap appears thinned. Key as in Fig. 5.13a.

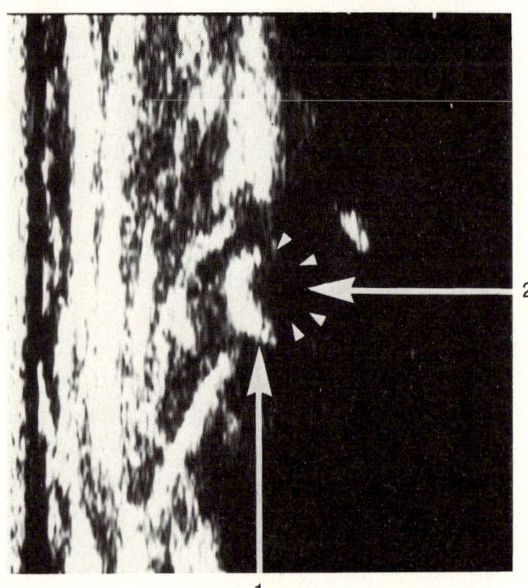

Fig. 5.14. Sonogram of a right hip joint with the half-moon phenomenon.

1 Lateral circumference of the femoral capital ossification centre
2 Invisible part of the ossification centre in the acoustic shadow

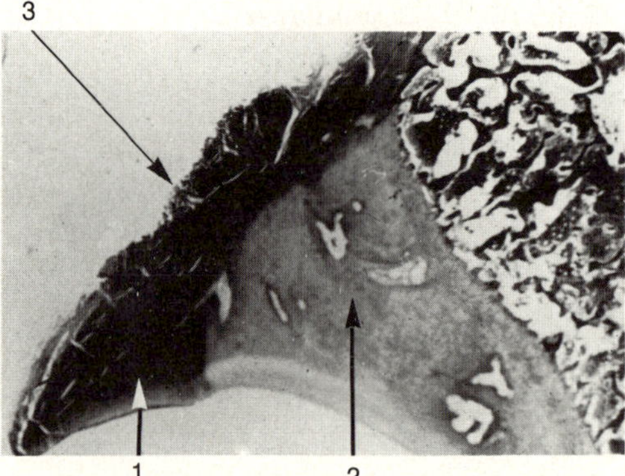

Fig. 5.15. Histological cut through the cartilaginous and bony parts of the acetabulum of a right hip.

1 Acetabular labrum
2 Acetabular roof preformed in hyaline cartilage
3 Joint capsule and perichondrium

5.3.3 The acetabular labrum

This forms a ring surrounding the acetabular roof, the free edge of which projects into the joint space. The ultrasound beam cuts it radially and produces a triangular echogenic shape. The variation in individual sizes of the circular band of the labrum is well-known from the procedure of implantation of total endoprostheses: it may be very wide or one may only see only a thin margin of fibrous collagen.

The major anatomical characteristics of the labrum at sonography are:

a) It is always the echo (or 'knot of echoes') which lies inferolateral to the echo gap in the hyaline part of the acetabular roof on the inside of the joint capsule.

b) It always lies inferolateral to the perichondrial gap (Figs. 5.12, 5.13).

c) It always maintains contact with the femoral head, even in the presence of gross dysplasia.

d) It can only lie in the position where the contour of the femoral head diverges from the joint capsule. This definition is particularly important in type IIIb hips (discussed later in chapter 11), in which the structure of the acetabular rim shows the same echogenicity as the labrum.

5.3.4 Questions of sonographic nomenclature

Unfortunately the nomenclature for the components of the acetabular roof is not unified. The concept of 'limbus' is too inexact for ultrasound diagnosis. Sometimes 'limbus' is used to mean the whole of the non-ossified parts of the acetabular roof (the labrum and the cartilaginous part of the roof). On the other hand, it has also been used to mean only the labrum, or only that part of the roof preformed in cartilage. We do not advocate the use of this term. Sonographically the cartilaginous acetabular roof (the cartilaginous roof or cartilaginous rim) and the acetabular labrum should be distinguished on the grounds of their differing echogenicity and their different behaviour during the process of dislocation.

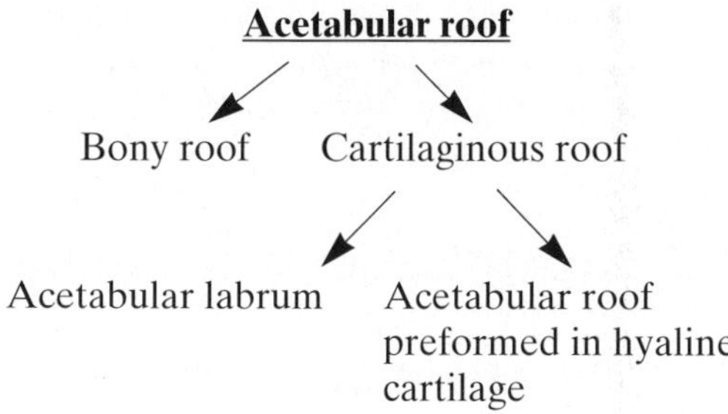

5.4 The floor of the acetabulum

When the ultrasound beam is directed in the coronal plane three typical layers of echogenicity can be made out, corresponding to the anatomical findings described in § 4.1.2. As expected, where the ultrasound beam strikes the bony parts, there is a strong echo, but where it meets the hyaline parts of the triradiate cartilage an echo gap can be found (Fig. 5.10).

5.4.1 The so-called 'fluid film'

In most cases the femoral head lies so close against the cartilaginous acetabular roof that the narrow joint space cannot be demonstrated sonographically. However in some sonograms a faint bow-shaped echo stripe, the so-called *'fluid film'*, can be seen at the border between the femoral head and the hyaline cartilaginous acetabular roof. Whether it is really caused by joint fluid or by a vacuum phenomenon is a moot point. Obviously if there are small physiological incongruencies in the movement of the hip this can lead to slight dehiscence of the joint surfaces which may be responsible. If the 'fluid film' is seen then the hyaline femoral head can be separated from its hyaline roofing so that the whole of the upper part of the circumference of the femoral head is demonstrated (Fig. 5.17).

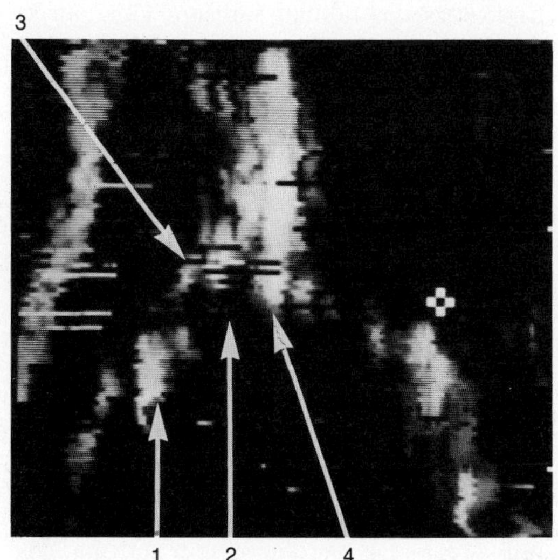

Fig. 5.16. Sonogram (enlarged) of the area of the right acetabular roof similar to the section in figure 5.15.

1 Acetabular labrum
2 Acetabular roof preformed in cartilage
3 Joint capsule and perichondrium
4 Bony acetabular rim

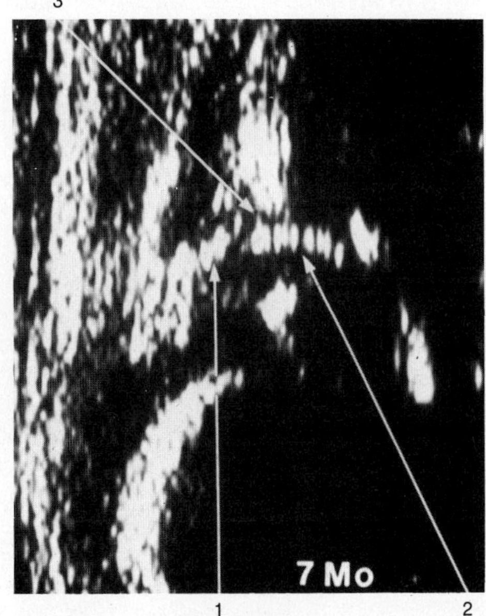

Fig. 5.17. Liquid film. The line of separation between the cartilaginous femoral head and the cartilaginous acetabular roof (the joint space).

1 Labrum
2 Joint space
3 Bony rim

However a second phenomenon may also be partly responsible for the sonographic distinction of the femoral head from its cartilaginous acetabular roof: histological examination shows that the *peripheral areas of hyaline cartilage* immediately subjacent to the joint surface on both the acetabular and the femoral sides are different from the remainder of the hyaline cartilage in the hip (Fig. 5.15). These internal 'borders' may also be implicated in the sonographic borderline separating the femoral head from the acetabular cartilage.

5.4.2 The ligament of the head of the femur

The structures of the ligament of the head of the femur which lie in the depths of the acetabular fossa and run into the fovea centralis should not be confused with the inferior border of the iliac bone. When the femoral head is rotated the echo of the fovea centra-

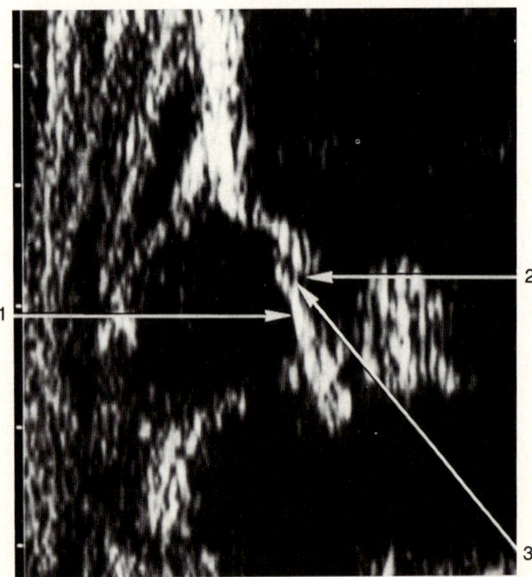

Fig. 5.18. Ligament of the head of the femur. The ligament (1) is strongly echogenic and should not be mistaken in its proximal part with the inferior border of the iliac bone (2). Between them lies the echo-poor zone of the tissue of the acetabular fossa (3)

lis lying lateral to the iliac bone move with it whereas the inferior border of the iliac bone remains stationary (Fig. 5.18).

5.5 Identification of anatomy at ultrasound: the standard situation

Recognition of the anatomical elements is paramount in ultrasound diagnosis of the hip joint. Difficulties in interpretation of the sonogram are particularly prone to arise in pathological cases, and unfortunately the images taken to document such cases are also often of limited value, so that important reference points on the acetabular roof are difficult to recognise.

It is therefore absolutely necessary to proceed systematically and identify the various structures in a clearly-defined order. These anatomical relationships do not in principle alter in any way even when the hip is dislocated (see also § 11.1).

The single most important structure to find is the acetabular labrum. This can be done reliably by identification of the *standard situation*.

The structure that acts as the principal guide is the strongly echogenic osteochondral junction on the femoral neck. This simplifies the search for the echo 'hole' that corresponds to the femoral head. After the identification of these structures, the echogenic connective tissue fold can be identified and confusion with the acetabular labrum prevented. Following the joint capsule *from lateral to medial around the circumference of the femoral head* from the tissue fold, the order of the structures encountered does not alter, and the first important one reached is the acetabular labrum. The next structure that encloses the labrum on its medial side is the cartilaginous rim of the acetabular roof, followed by the bony acetabular roof and the descending limb of the ilium. These are summarised in Table 5.1.

An accurate anatomical diagnosis allows for a correct second step in the process of

Table 5.1. The 'standard situation': the order of structures identifiable around the circumference of the femoral head:

Lateral ↓ ↓ Medial	Connective-tissue fold Acetabular labrum Cartilaginous acetabular roof Bony acetabular roof (including the bony rim and the inferior tip of the iliac bone)

interpretation, which is a rigorous description of the findings. This is discussed further in chapter 10, and includes notes on the bony formation, the contour of the rim, and the cartilaginous acetabular roof.

5.6 Practical procedure in difficult cases

5.6.1 Identification of the circumference of the femoral head

We have found that an inexperienced examiner may have difficulty in orientating himself in some difficult and highly pathological cases, and, as noted above, the hard copy may also be poor. We would like therefore to give some tips and tricks that can help to avoid mistakes and wrong diagnoses in the interpretation of the hip sonogram.

Our experience has shown that mistakes are usually caused by incorrect identification of anatomical structures on the sonogram. This is why it is absolutely necessary to proceed systematically.

A worthwhile simple trick is to place the ball of your thumb on the image of the femoral head and to follow the border of the femoral head around the thumb from the lateral to the superomedial side. On the circumference must now be found the standard situation, irrespective of the pathological state of the hip, and the identification of the acetabular labrum, the cartilage and the bony rim can be made. You will also easily see the extent of the bony roof covering of the femoral head – that is, whether the cartilaginous femoral head is covered with bone only in its medial third, or up to half or even two thirds.

5.6.2 Misidentification of the bony rim and acetabular labrum

This method of showing up the roundness of the hyaline femoral head also helps considerably the search for the point defined as the *bony rim* (see chapter 7) even if (as in highly pathological cases) the bony formation approximates almost to a sloping plane. Identification of the transitional point on a dysplastic acetabular roof from concavity to convexity as an equivalent to the "rim" becomes much more successful this way. This prevents the bony rim from being localised too far cranially. Watch out for this – in dislocated hips the bony rim is always found medio-caudal to the femoral head.

Difficulties in anatomical identification are typical of Type IIIb hips. Because of the echogenicity of the acetabular roof, in unfavourable cases the equally echogenic labrum and the cartilaginous rim may be impossible to differentiate from each other. In such cases the labrum lying peripherally or laterally may be mistaken for the bony rim. If such a structure is seen which is thought to be the bony rim, then even further peripherally around the circumference of the femoral head should be found the echo gap of the hyaline cartilaginous rim with the labrum lying peripherally to that. These structures however will be missing if this classical mistake has been made. If the standard situation is carefully observed: (1) labrum, (2) cartilage, (3) bone, then this mistake cannot happen.

Even when in pathological cases the labrum cannot be demonstrated as a clear echo, it is mandatory to localise it by aid of the nearby structures. The most common mistake in this connection is to identify the proximal perichondrium as the labrum. This mistake can be avoided by noting the topographical relationship between the proximal perichondrium, the perichondrial gap and the femoral head (Graf and Schuler 1986a).

The labrum may also be confused with the connective-tissue fold, which lies further laterally around the circumference of the femoral head.

Key points

- Much of the hip joint is cartilaginous at birth. The cartilaginous femoral head is separated from the bony diaphysis of the femoral shaft by the osteochondral junction.

- The acetabular roof can be seen to consist of cartilaginous and bony parts. The term 'limbus' is misleading.

- The acetabular labrum has typical anatomical relationships and is a particularly important structure to localise correctly.

- The osseous rim is defined as the point of transition on the acetabular roof from concavity to convexity.

- The femoral capital ossification centre causes progressive obscuration of the base of the acetabulum as it grows, and has an unreliable shape and position.

- Mistakes in anatomical diagnosis can be avoided by a strictly standardised procedure, progressing around the circumference of the femoral head. This is known as the standard situation.

6.1 Dividing hip joints into sonographic types

The term 'hip dysplasia' actually only encompasses disturbances of growth of the hip socket, and so diagnosis and classification of dysplasia can be made by reference to this area alone. However, the femoral head and socket mutually influence each other as a dynamic system, and the femoral head has a profound effect upon the development of the acetabulum during the process of dislocation. The normal and abnormal development of the whole of the hip can be described in terms of these underlying concepts.

In practice it is first of all wise to familiarise oneself with a normal completely mature (type I) hip, so that any departure from this norm becomes immediately apparent. This means that the examiner can usually immediately assign the correct value to a hip from the monitor, even in dynamic examinations; remember that diagnosis is facilitated by viewing the image as though looking at an AP radiograph of a right hip (see chapter 2).

6.1.1 Type I (Fig. 6.1 a–c)

This type of hip corresponds to a mature joint. A healthy joint exists both clinically and radiologically. The formation of the bony roof is good. The bony rim is angulated and well contoured. The cartilaginous acetabular roof consisting of the hyaline cartilaginous roof and the acetabular labrum is drawn downwards and outwards over the femoral head and clasps or overlaps it well.

Sonographic structure of the hyaline cartilaginous acetabular roof is echo-poor (the echo gap).

In many cases the bony rim as described above is arrow-shaped, angular and sharply bordered (Fig. 6.1b). However, a slight rounding-off of the edges may also be seen and is quite permissible (Fig. 6.1c). The shape of the bony roof still corresponds to a mature and correctly roofed hip, and the relationships of the angles which will be discussed later do not alter: note that we can also often see similar variations on the plain

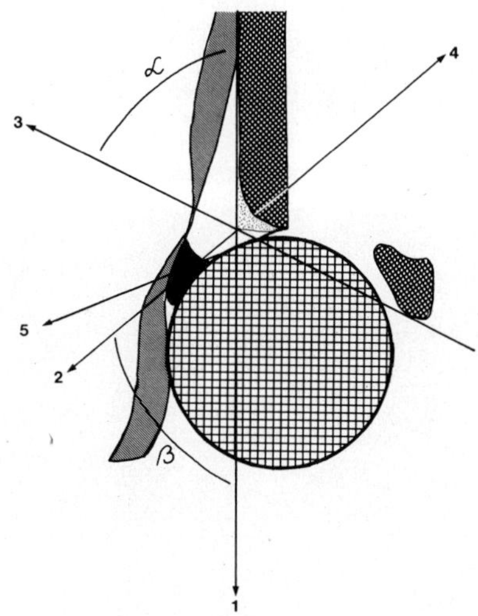

Fig. 6.1a. Schematic drawing of a hip joint, type I, with a sharp bony rim tailing off distally.

1 Soft tissue fold
2 Cartilage roof line
3 Bony roof line
4 'Tailing-off' (blunt) bony rim
5 Cartilaginous roof line as it would be with a blunt bony rim
   α Bony angle
   β Cartilaginous angle

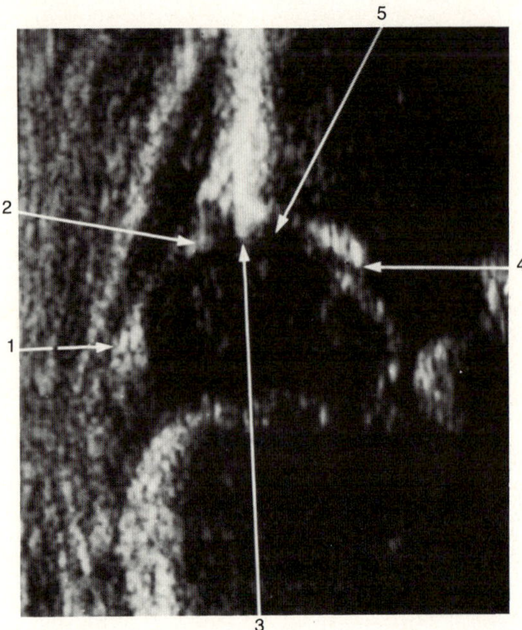

Fig. 6.1b. Sonogram of a two-month-old baby, right hip: type I. Arrow-shaped, well-contoured bony rim.

1 Joint capsule
2 Acetabular labrum
3 Well-contoured, sharp bony rim
4 Ilium
5 Acoustic shadow behind the bony rim

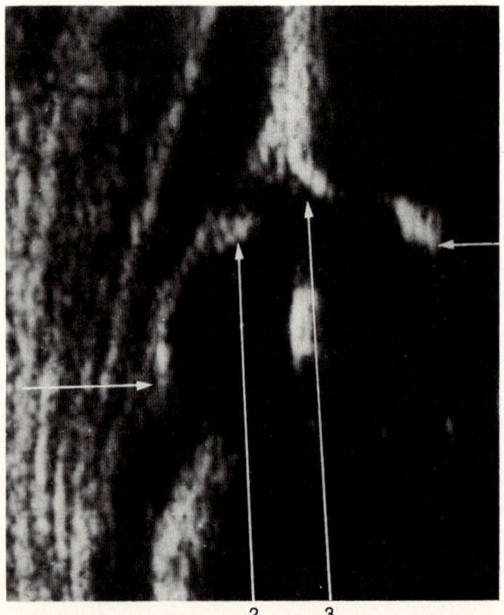

radiograph, without there being any dysplasia present. For this minimally rounded acetabular rim, the concept of a 'tailing-off' or 'blunt' rim has been adopted.

6.1.2 Type II (Fig. 6.2 a–g)

The bony roof is deficient, the bony rim is more or less rounded, and the bony socket appears to be dysplastic. On the other hand the cartilaginous parts of the acetabular roof continue to form a complete covering, so that the overhanging cartilage appears widened but still overlaps the femoral head.

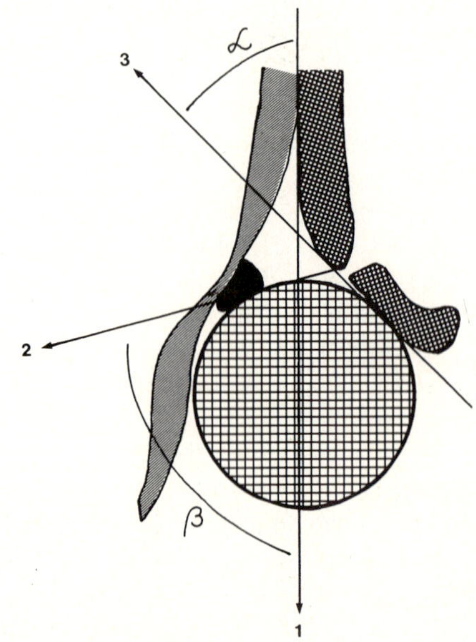

Fig. 6.2a. Schematic drawing of a right hip. Type II. The total roofing of the acetabulum is adequate. The relationships between the cartilaginous and bony parts of the acetabular roof are disturbed in favour of the cartilage.

1 Baseline
2 Cartilage roof line
3 Bony roof line
  α Bony angle
  β Cartilaginous angle

◄ **Fig. 6.1c.** Hip type I, with a blunt bony rim (3). Key as in Figure 6.1b. Description: Good bony formation with a blunted bony rim

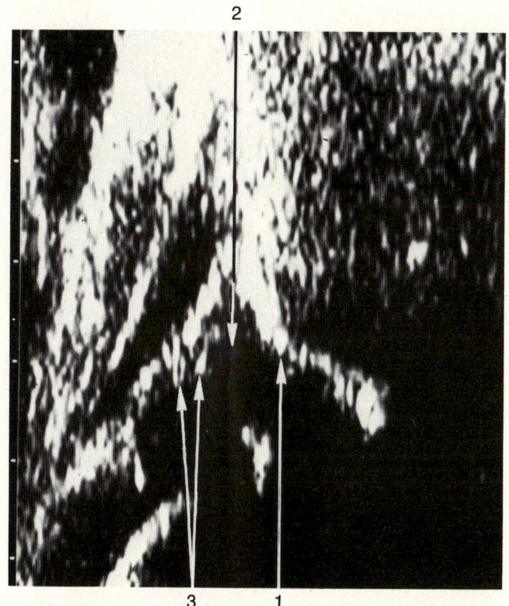

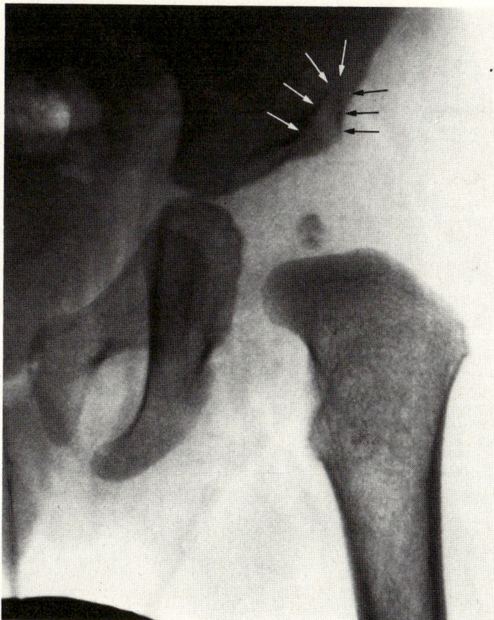

Fig. 6.2b. Left hip, nine-month-old child. The bony rim is rounded, and the bony formation is lacking. The cartilaginous rim overlaps the femoral head widely: type II. The section runs through the bony rim defect in Figure 6.2c (sonogram projected as for a right hip).

1 Transitional zone of the bony rim
2 Cartilaginous rim
3 Acetabular labrum

Fig. 6.2c. Left hip dysplasia. There is a defect in the rim between the front and rear portions of the acetabular roof, marked with arrows

The hyaline acetabular roof is still echo-poor. Because adequate ossification of the cartilaginous part of the roof has not yet occurred this type of hip is said to be suffering from *delayed ossification*. The congruity of the joint is maintained.

6.1.3 Type III (Figs. 6.3 and 6.4)

If the flattening of the bony overhang continues to increase, then the load-bearing, firm bony roofing of the femoral head fails. The total pressure of the femoral head pressing cranially overloads the cartilaginous acetabular roof and it begins to bend cranially and laterally. We call this type of hip with superolateral distortion of the cartilaginous acetabular roof a *type III* hip.

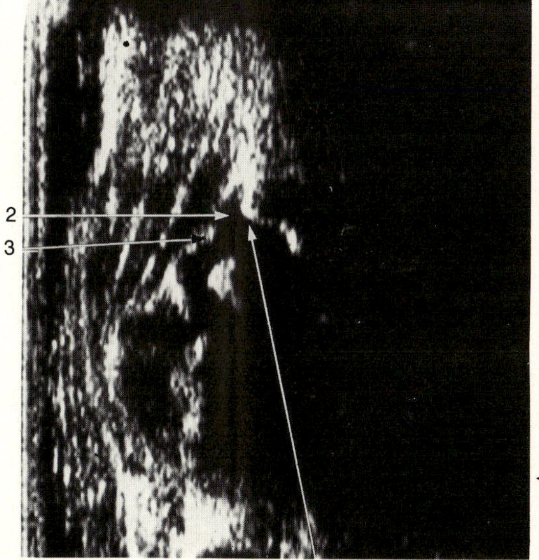

◄ **Fig. 6.2d.** The bony rim (1) is round, bony formation is adequate, and is compensated for by the cartilaginous rim which widely overlaps the femoral head (2). Acetabular labrum (3). Type II hip

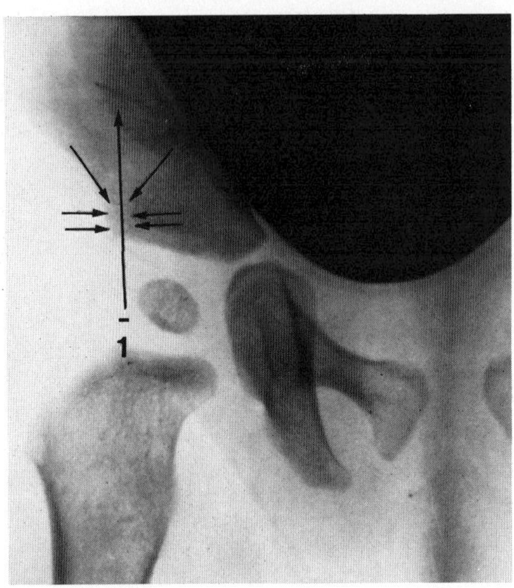

Fig. 6.2e. Radiograph to Figure 6.2d. The defect in the rim is marked with arrows. The standard plane runs through the middle of the acetabular roof

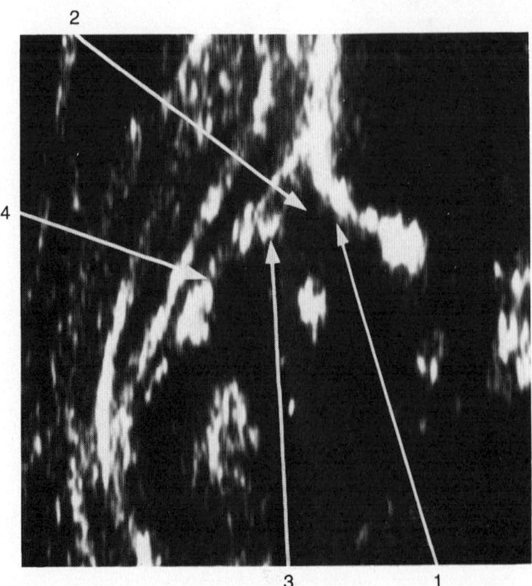

Fig. 6.2f. Three-month-old joint, deficient bony formation.

1 Bony rim markedly rounded
2 Cartilaginous rim very wide, but overlapping the femoral head
3 Acetabular labrum
4 Joint capsule

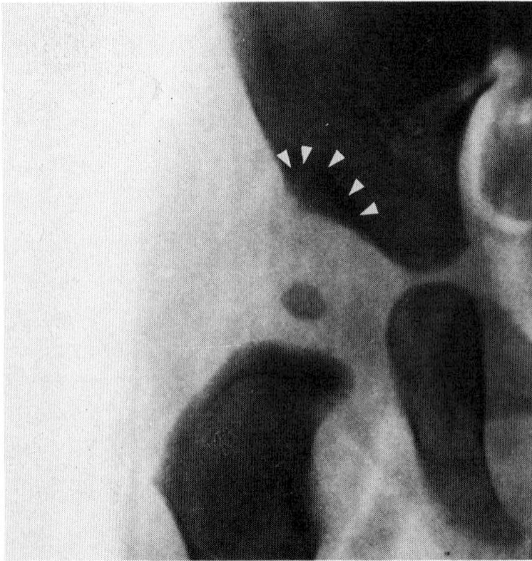

Fig. 6.2g. Radiograph corresponding to Figure 6.2f. Severe rim defect, with only the posterior part of the rim of the hip socket well developed. The defect in the rim is marked with arrows. This defect is compensated for by cartilage

Type III hips may be subdivided according to the effect of the pressure upon the hyaline roof cartilage:

In *type IIIa* hips, the structure of the cartilage remains normal and echo-poor (Fig. 6.3a and 6.3b). Distinction of type IIIa hips from type D hips is dealt with in chapter 8.

In *type IIIb* hips, the pressure has risen so high that it induces histological change in the hyaline cartilage. The regular cartilaginous architecture is lost, particularly in the border between the cartilage and adjoining layer of bone (Fig. 4.6). Collagen fibrils lying in the cartilage are normally masked by intercellular cement and are invisible on light microscopy. These become unmasked and microscopically visible. Because of this disturbance of structure, the typical echo-poor structure of the hyaline cartilaginous roof is lost and the *cartilage becomes echogenic* (Fig. 6.4a). These remarkable histological changes are clearly visible in Figure

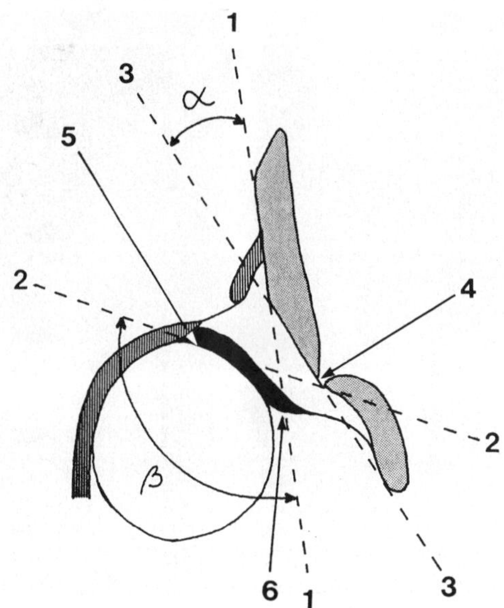

Fig. 6.3a. Schematic drawing of the right hip. Type IIIa (without disturbance of the histological structure, as the cartilaginous part of the acetabular roof is echo-poor).

1 Base line
2 Cartilage roof line
3 Acetabular roof line
  α Bony angle
  β Cartilaginous angle
4 Transitional point
5 Labrum elongated cranially
6 Hypomochlion

Fig. 6.3b. Neonatal hip joint corresponding to Figure 6.3c and 6.3d. The bony formation is poor. The bony rim is flat, the cartilaginous acetabular roof is compressed cranially and echopoor. Type IIIa.

1 Joint capsule
2 Acetabular labrum
3 Bony rim

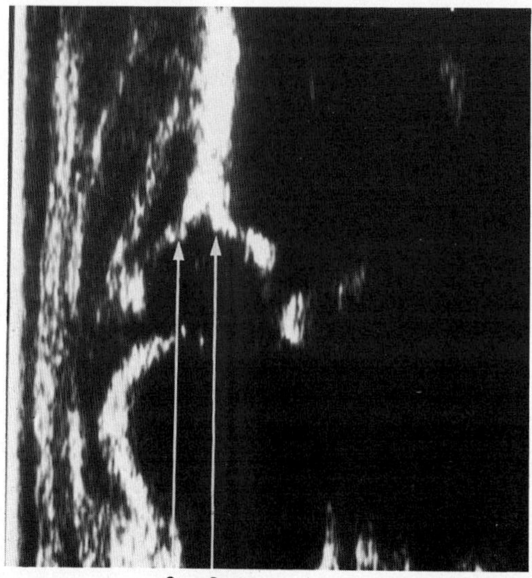

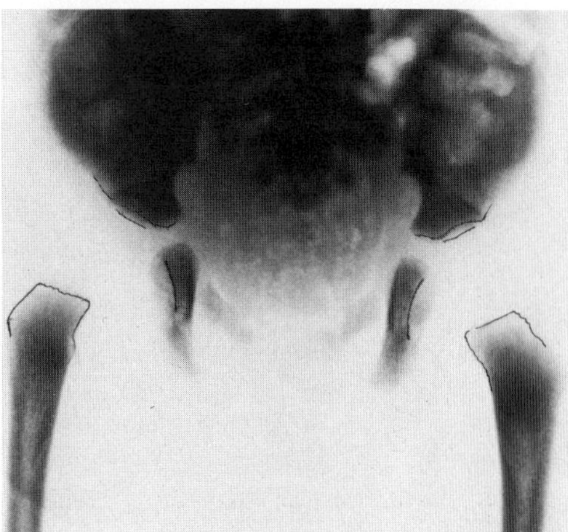

Fig. 6.3d. Radiograph to Figure 6.3b, c. The right hip joint is dislocated

◀ **Fig. 6.3c.** The bony formation is good. The bony rim is sharply angulated, the cartilaginous part of the roof overlaps the femoral head. Type I (key as in Figure 6.3b)

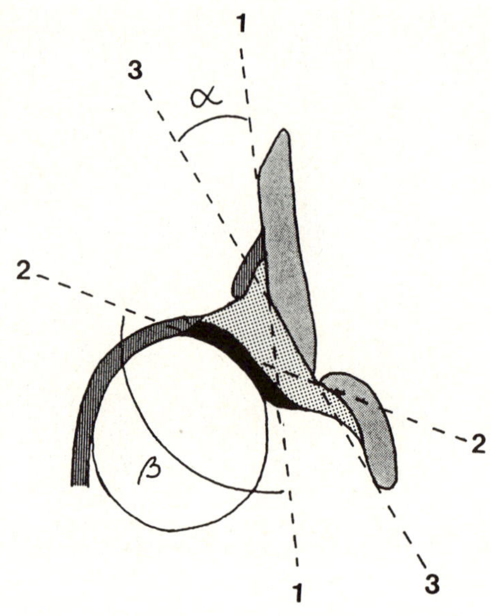

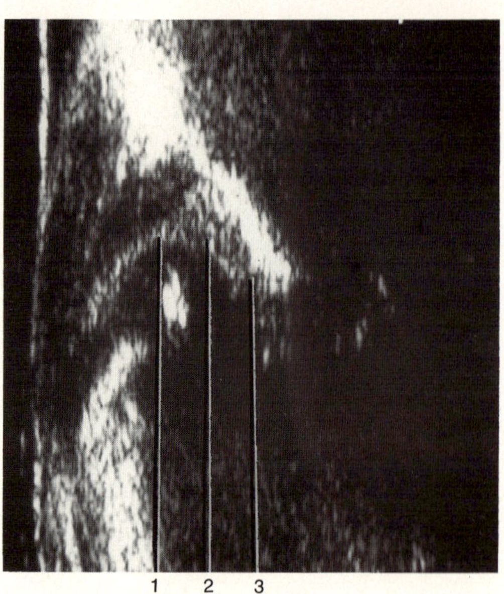

Fig. 6.4a. Right hip type IIIb schematic. The cartilage is altered by the pressure and has become echogenic. Key as in Figure 6.3a

Fig. 6.4b. Sonogram of the right hip. Six month old infant, with a clear increase in echogenicity (3) in the cartilaginous acetabular roof. The bony formation is grossly deficient, the bony rim is markedly rounded or flattened (2), the cartilaginous rim is echogenic, widened and squeezed against the acetabular labrum (1). The inferior rim of the ilium lies outwith the standard plane and cannot be seen

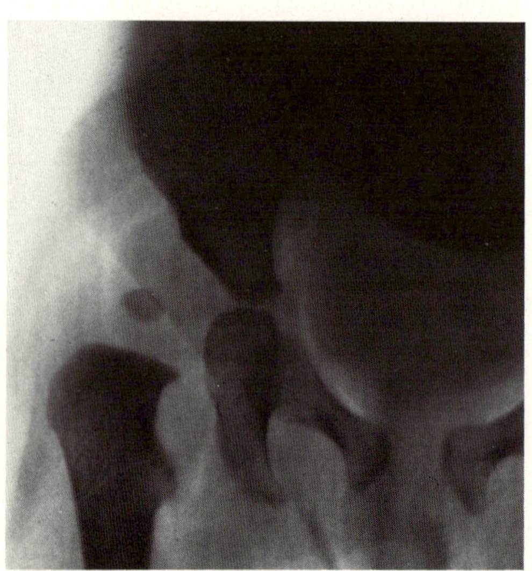

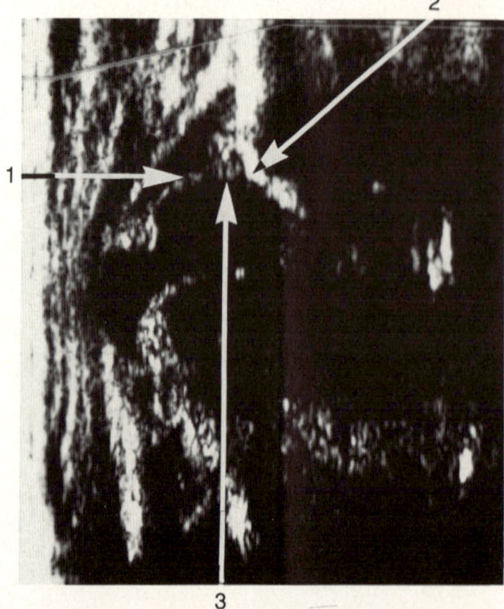

Fig. 6.4c. Radiograph to Figure 6.4a

Fig. 6.4d. Eight week old baby, right hip. Sonogram with the cartilaginous rim clearly compressed upwards and echogenic (3). The bony formation is deficient, the bony rim (2) is rounded, type IIIb. (1) Acetabular labrum

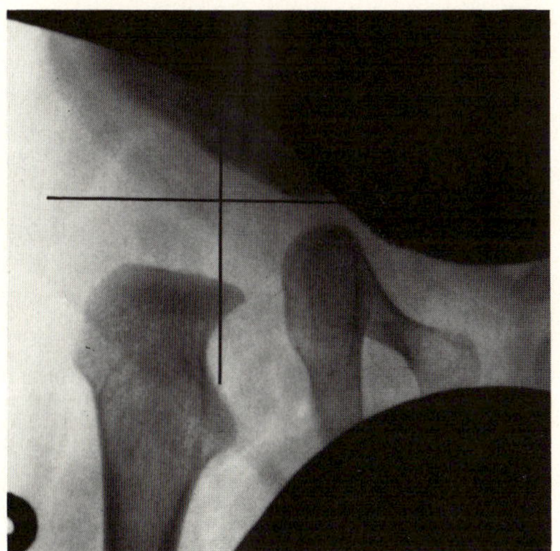

Fig. 6.4e. Radiograph to Figure 6.4d. The low grade of dislocation is noteworthy, as it gives a misleading impression of the real degree of the lesion. The acetabular cartilage is considerably damaged, as is shown at ultrasound

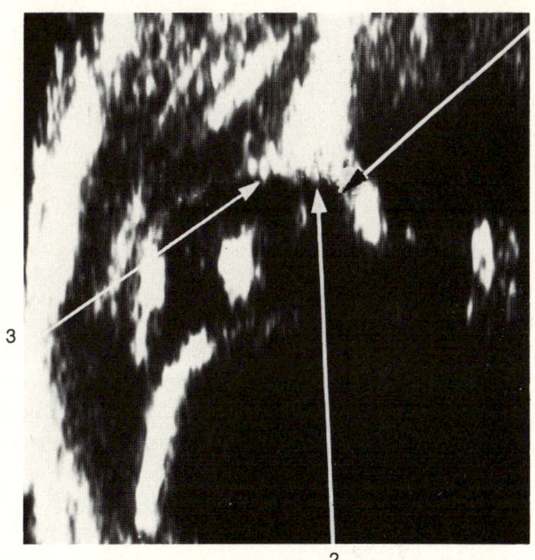

Fig. 6.5. Four month old right hip. Bony rim (1) is flat. The cartilaginous roof is wide, compressed and has a dense structure (2). Type IIIb. 3 = acetabular labrum

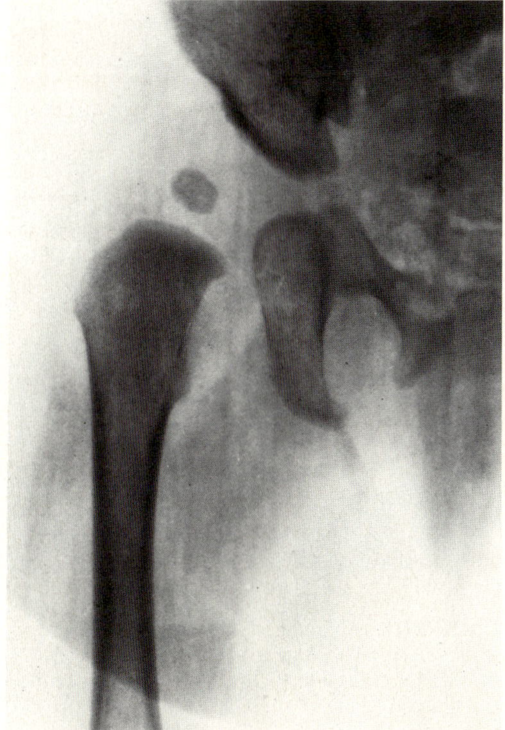

Fig. 6.6. Radiograph to Figure 6.5. There is only slight dislocation although sonographically considerable disturbance of the structure can already be found in the cartilaginous roof

4.13 and give a logical explanation for the sudden rise in echogenicity. (Radiographically type IIIa hips cannot be distinguished from type IIIb).

Type IIIb hips have a worse outlook than type IIIa hips. The first result of successful treatment of a type IIIb hip is a recovery of the sonographicaly echo-poor structure of the acetabular roof and effective transformation into a type IIIa hip. Only after this has happened, and further measures are taken to relieve the pressure on the acetabular roof, can the compressed and deformed cartilage reassume its normal configuration.

It is quite important to note that the type IIIb hip is not necessarily a 'high' dislocation (see Fig. 6.4b to e). Often the degree of dislocation is only slight, and the cartilage has been damaged rather than, as in a type IIIa hip, being stretched over the femoral head but retaining a relatively normal structure (Figs. 6.5, 6.6).

The femoral head is also exposed to raised pressure in this situation and the fact that its echogenicity does not increase is due to two causes:

1. The pressure is better distributed over the spherical surface.
2. Shearing forces as well as compressive forces are responsible for the deformation of the acetabular roof.

6.1.4 Type IV (Fig. 6.7a–d)

In this type the femoral head luxates superolaterally. However, unlike in the type III hip, the hyaline acetabular roof and its labrum are not pushed cranially but slide down and away from the femoral head in a mediocaudal direction and become compressed between the femoral head and the iliac bone. No acetabular cartilage can be seen between the femoral head and the iliac bone.

Using viewing planes similar to a conventional tomogram, the femoral head in the type IV hip can usually be localised among the soft tissues without problem. Only in favourable cases is it sometimes possible to see past the femoral neck and medially in to where the true acetabulum is to be seen filled with loose tissue (Fig. 6.7b).

There are important therapeutic complications arising out of this over and above those of type III hips. Manoeuvres to reduce the type IV joint are considerably more difficult than in the case of the type III joint, and the femoral head is more endangered. This is because of the constriction of the mouth of the acetabulum caused by the inwardly compressed cartilage. In general, sonographic typing of hip joints does not take into account the height of the dislocation, as this is a poor predictor of the outcome of therapy.

Note that a type IIIa hip does not have to pass through the IIIb stage on its way to

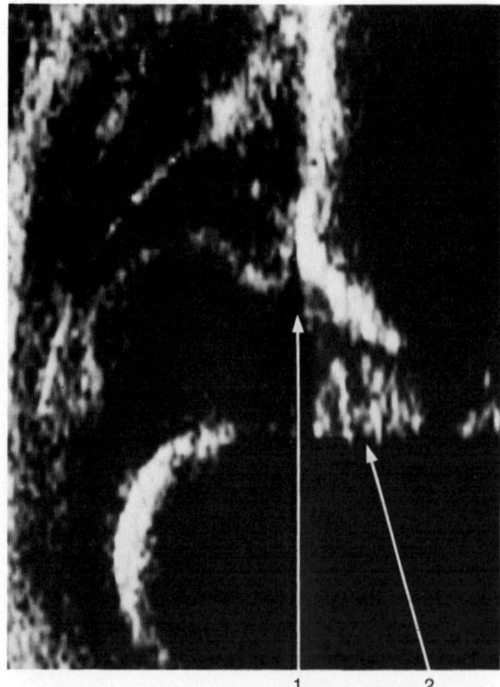

Fig. 6.7a. Figure 6.7aHip type IV, schematic. The femoral head has compressed the hyaline acetabular roof with its elongated acetabular labrum between itself and the bony socket.

1 Joint capsule ('hood-shaped')
2 Elongated and compressed labrum
3 Parts of the cartilaginous acetabular roof compressed medio-caudally, serving the dislocated femoral head as a 'hypomochlion'

Fig. 6.7b. Four-week-old hip joint, type IV. Sonogram corresponding with Figure 6.7a. The femoral head is clearly dislocated, more laterally than cranially. The cartilaginous roof is compressed between the femoral head and the lamellar bone (1). No cartilaginous roof can be seen cranial to the femoral head and outside the strip of joint capsule and perichondrium. In the depths of the acetabular fossa, several echoes represent the loose tissue of the vacant space (2)

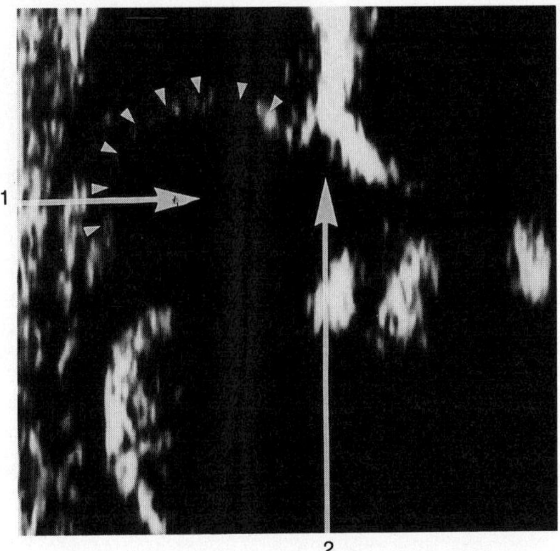

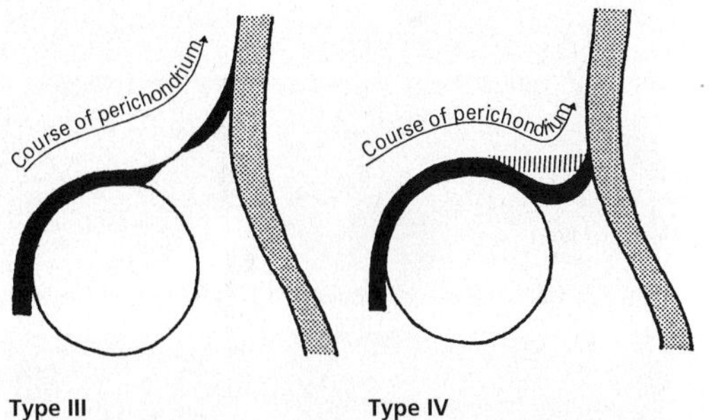

Fig. 6.7c. Four-week old hip joint. The femoral head (1) is dislocated. The 'hood' of capsule is clearly visible. The cartilaginous acetabular roof has been pressed caudally by the femoral head (2)

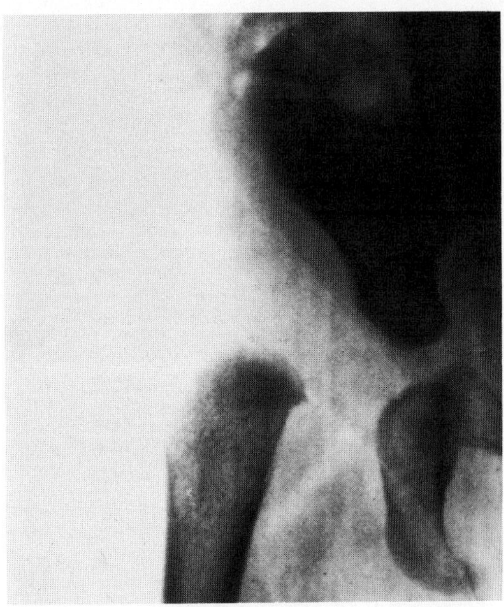

Fig. 6.7d. Radiograph to Figure 6.7c

Fig. 6.7e. Distinction between types III and IV hips by the direction and course of the perichondrium on the cartilaginous acetabular roof

becoming a type IV hip. Figures 6.8 and 6.9 show a hip at a transitional stage between IIIa and IV, with considerable dislocation. However, the echo texture of the acetabular roof is still normal. On the other hand, it is possible to show alterations in the structure of the cartilaginous acetabular roof in some cases of type IV hips, and this should be noted in addition to the basic typing. This group is particularly difficult to manage (Graf and Schuler, 1986). In a further number of type IV hips, the roof cartilage is hidden within the acetabulum and cannot be assessed at all.

6.1.5 Sonographic differentiation between types III and IV

Localisation of the labrum in the type IV hip is often difficult because of the high grade compression. Thus it is impractical to differentiate between type III and type IV hips by the localisation of the acetabular labrum. Instead, this is routinely done by observing the *course of the perichondrium* on the cartilage of the acetabular roof. This perichondrium acts as an indicator to show the direction and the degree to which the cartilage has been compressed: if the perichondrium is drawn cranially a type III is present, but if the perichondrium forms a trough between the femoral head and the acetabular roof or if it runs horizontally, a type IV hip is present (Figs. 6.7e, 6.10 and 6.11).

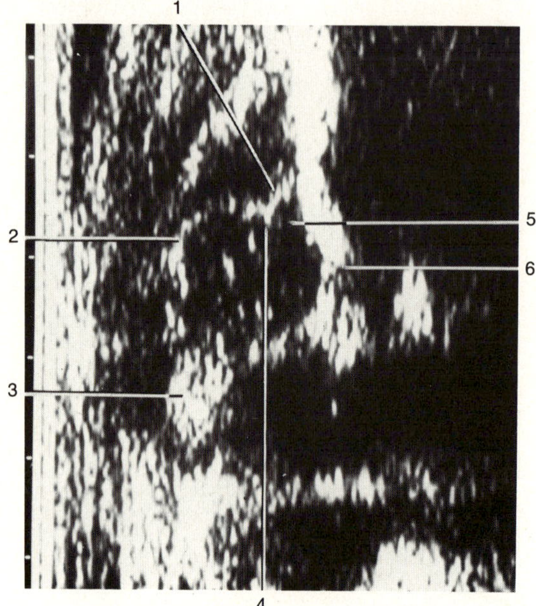

Fig. 6.8. Thirteen day old baby. The femoral head has started to squash the larger part of the acetabular roof cartilage between itself and the iliac wall. Only a small portion of the cartilage still lies cranial to the femoral head. The hip joint is on the border between type IIIa and type IV.

1 Perichondrium
2 Joint capsule
3 Osteochondral border
4 Labrum
5 Cartilaginous acetabular roof
6 Inferior tip of the iliac bone

6.2 The problem of the echogenic cartilaginous rim

6.2.1 The reference point

Naturally the amplification settings of the machine should be taken into account if one wants to differentiate between echo-poor and echogenic states of the cartilaginous acetabular rim. The ultrasound apparatus should be set so that the hyaline femoral head appears echo-poor or echo-free (see chapter 3). If the overall intensity or the depth gain control is set too high, it can lead to over-insonation of the picture and echoes can be clearly seen both in the hyaline femo-

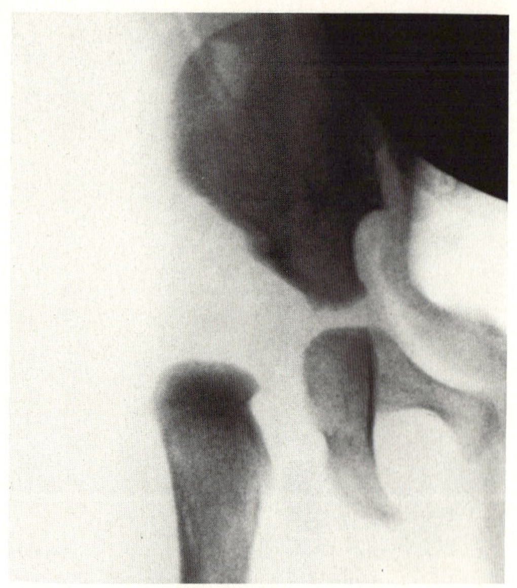

Fig. 6.9. Radiograph to Figure 6.9

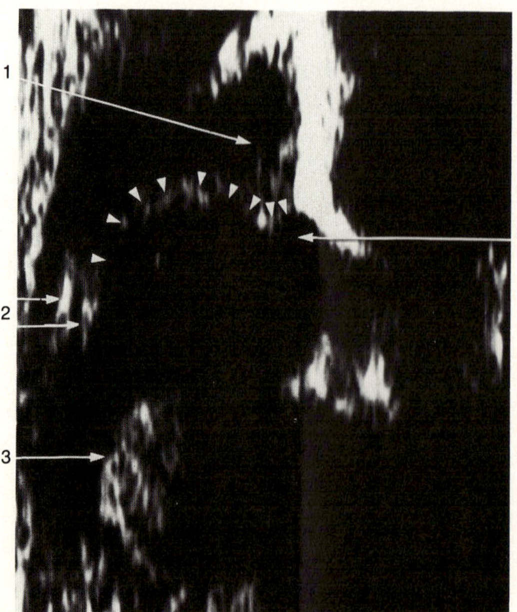

Fig. 6.10. Four week old hip joint, type IV. The cartilaginous acetabular roof (4) is jammed between the femoral head and the bone. The hood of capsule and the perichondrium are marked with arrow heads. The only structures to be found proximal to the joint capsule are:

1 Gluteus minimus muscle
2 Fold of connective tissue
3 Osteochondral border
4 Cartilaginous acetabular roof

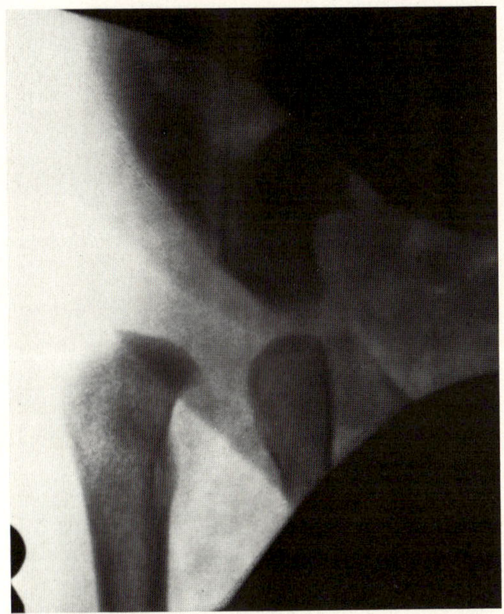

Fig. 6.11. Radiograph to Figure 6.10

ral head and in the cartilage of the acetabular roof. These can lead to a false impression that the acetabular roof has become hyperechogenic.

To avoid this, a reference point with a corresponding structure has to be found for comparison. This should lie immediately adjacent to the acetabulum and should be at the same depth, so that it undergoes the same degree of amplification. The *femoral head* lying immediately underneath the acetabulum fulfils all these criteria.

Echoes seen in the femoral head should thus be subtracted from any echoes present in the hyaline acetabular roof before any judgement is made as to the residual echogenicity of the roof, which in this special case amounts to histological classification.

Correct assessments are demonstrated in Figure 6.12a and 6.12b. Although in Figure 6.12a clear echoes and an apparent echoge-

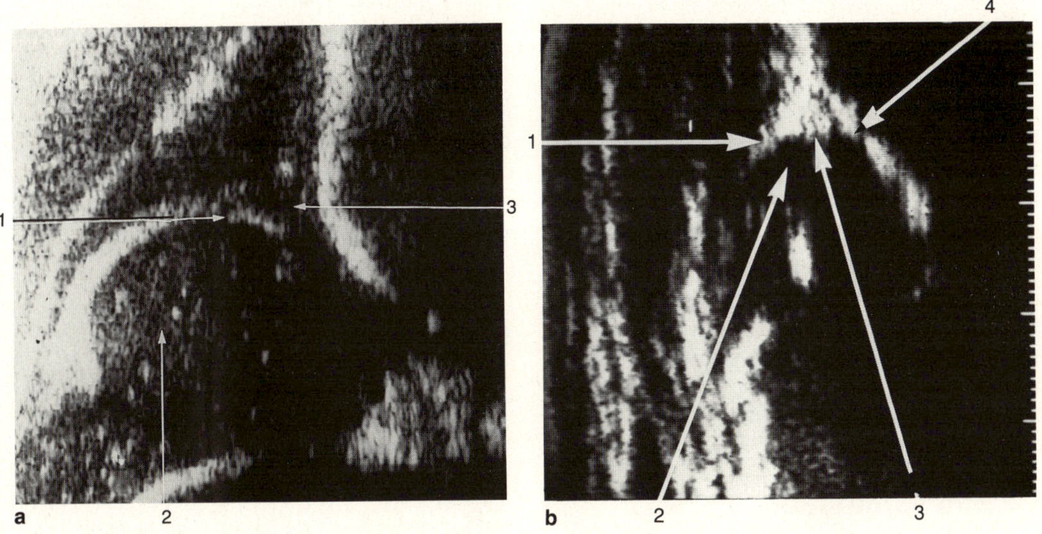

Fig. 6.12a, b. For comparison between Figure 6.12a and b, and Figure 6.12c and d.

1 Acetabular labrum
2 Cartilaginous femoral head
3 Cartilaginous acetabular roof
4 Transitional point equivalent to the bony rim

In Figure 6.12a, clear echoes are seen in the cartilaginous acetabular roof. Similar echoes are present in the femoral head (2) lying underneath it. If these echoes are 'subtracted' from the ones in the acetabular roof, the roof is seen to be relatively echo-free: type IIIa.

In Figure 6.12b, the cartilaginous acetabular roof (3) is clearly echogenic compared to the reference point of the femoral head (2): type IIIb

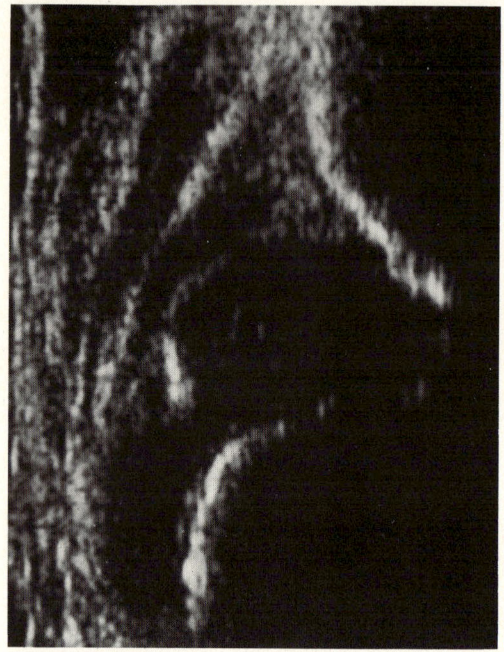

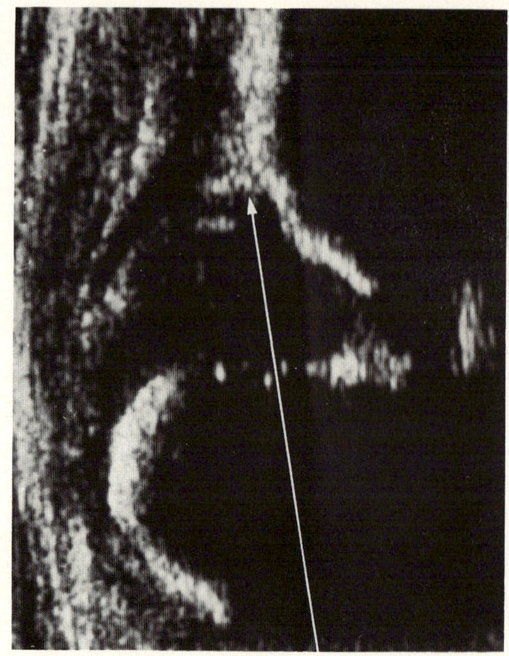

Fig. 6.12c. Type IIIb joint. The cartilaginous acetabular roof is completely echogenic compared with Figure 6.12d

Fig. 6.12d. Only the proximal part of the cartilaginous acetabular roof in the region of the perichondrial gap is echogenic (1), because of artefactual reverberation echoes. Type IIIa joint

nicity of the cartilaginous rim are seen, this hip should be allocated to type IIIa, as there are equally strong echoes in the femoral head: if these echoes are subtracted from those in the acetabulum, then the acetabular cartilage has to be regarded as echo-poor.

In Figure 6.12b the echoes visible in the deformed cartilaginous roof are clearly stronger than in the femoral head which lies underneath it and is almost echo-free – thus type IIIb.

6.2.2 Reverberation artefacts

The ultrasound wave can oscillate between the highly echogenic proximal perichondrium and the bony lamella lying immediately medial to it and which is equally strongly reflective, and this can lead to added echoes in this area. These echoes are artefacts and should not be confused with an alteration of the structure in the hyaline cartilage. Thus in principle the most superficial echoes in the

hyaline cartilage should not be used for determination of the structure; increased echogenicity in the hyaline cartilage should only be described when the whole cartilage is echogenic.

6.2.3 Pathological and physiological echogenicity

The cartilaginous part of the roof can be followed sonographically as it physiologically ossifies, the residual cartilage gradually waning in size as it does so. This is initially visible as a narrow slit running far cranially which progressively loses its 'echo gap' from cranial to caudal and becomes echogenic. With advancing maturity of the acetabular roof only a small U-shaped echo gap is visible around the bony rim, corresponding to the remains of the hyaline cartilage. This so-called physiological 'U' remains present in late examinations of the hip (Fig. 6.13a).

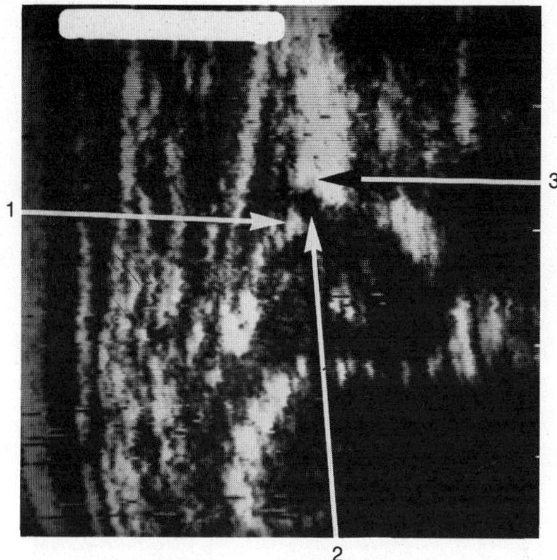

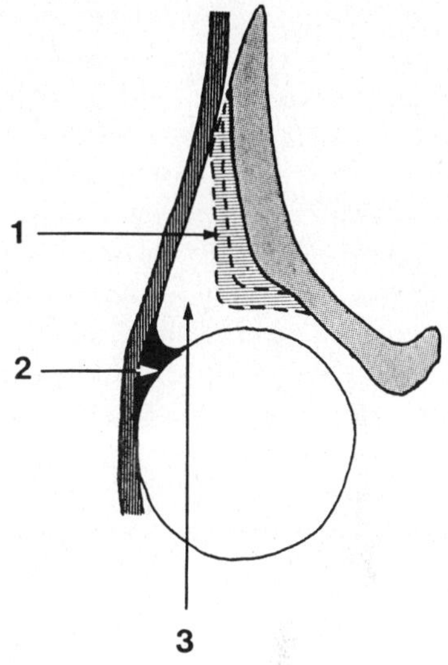

Fig. 6.13a. Matured hip, type I. Well-developed, angulated bony rim. The cartilaginous rim is narrow and grips the femoral head, and has a normal form and structure.

1 Acetabular labrum
2 Physiological 'U'
3 Cartilaginous rim, largely invaded by ossification

Fig. 6.13b. Schematic drawing to show secondary ossification.

1 Echogenicity increasing from proximal to distal
2 Acetabular labrum
3 Part of the cartilaginous acetabular roof not yet ossified

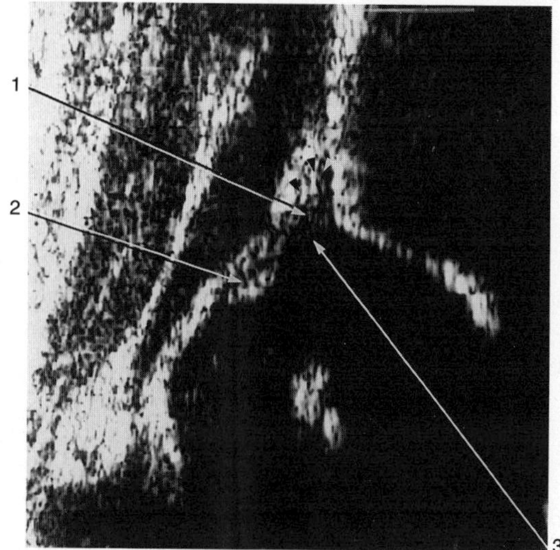

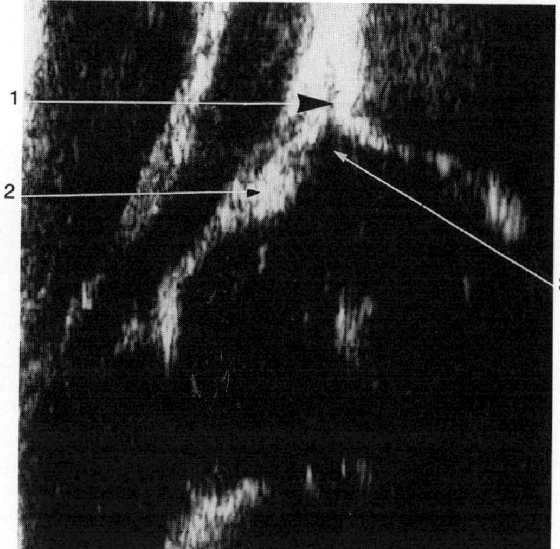

Fig. 6.13c. Nine month old patient with defective bony formation and a widely overlapping but not compressed cartilaginous acetabular roof. The wide cartilaginous promontory is already echogenic in its proximal part (1, marked with arrow). Key as in Fig.6.13b

Fig. 6.13d. The same patient as in Fig.6.13c two months later. Secondary ossification. The contours of the bony process have advanced, the bony formation is clearly better, and compared with Fig.6.13c the cartilaginous process rim clearly narrower and becoming consumed. Key as in Fig.6.13b

These physiologically dense cartilaginous rims with their remaining small echo gap should not be confused with hips in which the acetabula are unossified but showing a disturbance of structure (which is pathological). The distinction between 'disturbance of structure' and 'secondary ossification' is only possible through differentiating between centred and dislocated hips. It is known from follow-up of radiographs that development of the acetabular rim (i.e., physiological secondary ossification) is only possible with properly located femoral heads.

A single patient may show two hips in each of which the angles are normally matured, but in which the hyaline cartilage has been encroached upon by the advancing bone to differing extents. One hip may then be said to be further advanced than the other on the grounds of the ossification of its cartilage.

A particular case is that of the type II hips. Even when they continue to show insufficient total bony roofing, the inception of secondary ossification can lead to the development of an angular contour in the bony rim as a sign of growth in the acetabular roof.

A similar early change can be seen on the radiograph even when the angular relationships are still dysplastic. This *physiological ossification* does not always mean that the socket is already mature, but can always be seen as a favourable prognostic sign (Fig. 6.13b–d).

A phenomenon noted in § 5.2.3 with regard to the femoral head is also seen here in the acetabular roof: the echoes of this physiological ossification develop on the sonogram some 4–6 weeks before the accompanying calcification on the plain radiograph. Thus, the secondary ossification may cause a hip to appear less dysplastic on the sonogram than it does on the radiograph.

The remodelling of the cartilaginous acetabular roof does not happen in toto but can be patchy and fragmented. In one and the same acetabular roof, areas with and without echogenicity can be found in different sections. Complete remodelling in IIIb hip joints is only found in rare cases. If this is not the case the examiner has to base his judgement upon whether or more or less than half of the acetabular roof shows structural disturbance.

Key points

- Dysplasia of the hip is confined to dysplasia of the acetabulum and the effect of the femoral head upon it.

- Hips may be divided into basic types according to:
  The degree of coverage provided by the acetabular roof,
  The degree to which the acetabular roof is ossified,
  Any change in echogenicity induced in the roof cartilage by the pressure of the femoral head,
  Whether or not the femoral head is dislocated,
  The direction in which the acetabular roof is compressed by a dislocated head.

- Echogenicity of a cartilaginous roof can only be recognised by comparison with the femoral head lying underneath it.

- Echogenicity may also be mimicked by reverberation artefacts.

- There are two important causes of increased echogenicity in the acetabular roof: pathological alteration of structure, and physiological secondary ossification. These can be distinguished by noting whether or not the femoral head is dislocated.

7 Standard levels, measurement technique and measurement errors

7.1 The standard section

In order to carry out a reproducible quantification of the acetabular roof it is necessary to establish a standard measurement plane.

7.1.1 Variations in planes of section

It is possible to take a variety of sections through the acetabulum (Fig. 7.1 and 7.2):

1. *Rotated* sections (cuts a_1 and a_2). These sections are rotated about the central (transverse) axis of the acetabulum, and pass obliquely down from supero-anterior to infero-posterior or from supero-posterior to infero-anterior. It is obvious that the dorsal part of the bony roof of the acetabulum is in general very well developed, the middle and load bearing part is moderately well covered, while the anterior parts give only a rather slight roofing to the femoral head (Fig. 7.1). This peculiarity implies that if a cut is taken through the acetabulum running through the dorsal part of the edge of the socket (cut a_2 in Fig. 7.1), a relatively good bony roofing is always shown. Cuts through the middle (b_2 in Fig. 7.1) and anterior (a_1 in Fig. 7.1) parts of the socket show progressively poorer degrees of roofing.

2. *Tilted* sections. Such sections may be tilted forwards or backwards around a supero-inferior axis by anything up to 45°. The acetabulum is cut through at an angle. Such tipping of the transducer causes measurement errors which make the resulting images useless.

3. *True coronal* sections (section b in Fig. 7.1 and 7.2). The optimal compromise be-

tween good (section a_2) and bad (a_1) proportions of the acetabular roof is provided by the middle section (b_2 in Fig. 7.1). These

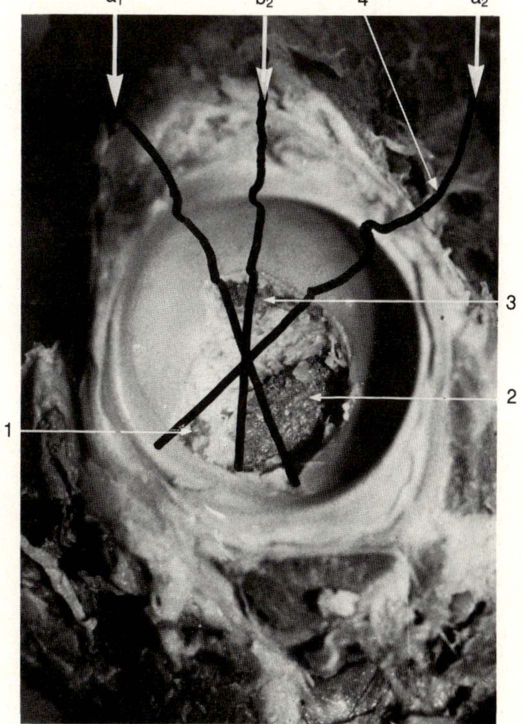

Fig. 7.1. View of left acetabulum. Three planes of section through the acetabular fossa.

a_1 This section cuts the front of the acetabular roof

b_2 Exact coronal section

a_2 This cut runs away over the humped posterior part of the acetabular roof and into the concavity (4) of the gluteal fossa.

1 Pubic bone

2 Ischial bone

3 Iliac bone

are laid in the coronal plane of the body through the acetabular fossa.

However it is necessary to define *three reference points* to define a plane in space. Along section b_2, the standard three points are:

a) The inferior tip of the iliac bone in the depth of the acetabular fossa,
b) The flat edge of the iliac wing, which is used to define the middle of the acetabular roof (see below),
c) The acetabular labrum.

7.2 The anatomical landmarks

7.2.1 The inferior border of the iliac bone and the acetabular floor

The acetabulum appears more or less rounded on sonography and, since its centre cannot be found mathematically, the so-called *lower border of the iliac bone* in the acetabular fossa serves as a marker point for the middle of the acetabulum. This inferior rim is formed by the part of the iliac bone in the acetabular fossa which is not covered by the lunate fascia (Fig. 7.1). Demonstration of this rim as a strong echo is a sign that the cut has been successfully taken through load bearing part of the acetabulum in sector A, and is the first requirement for establishing the standard plane.

Because of the particular shape of the curvature of the ilium, its inferior border cannot be demonstrated ventral to sections a_1 or dorsal to a_2. On these more peripheral sections, the base of the ilium is cut through tangentially and tails away medially on the sonogram (compare Figs. 7.1 and 7.5).

The sonographic planes can be classified even more exactly when the various anatomical structures of the acetabular fossa are taken into account. In this region, the floor of the socket is composed of three layers (Figs. 7.2, 7.3), as described in chapter 4.

1. The deep or medial layer, composed of the iliac bone cranially, dorsally of the ischial bone and ventrally from small parts of the pubic bone. All these bones are bound together in the triradiate cartilage (Fig. 7.1).

2. The intermediate layer, made up of the fat and connective tissue that invest the acetabular fossa.

3. The lateral (superficial) layer, consisting of the ligament of the head of the femur.

Echoes from all these structures may be seen on appropriate sonographic sections. If one follows the various sections from cranial to caudal, the following can be established (compare Fig. 7.2 with 7.3):

Section a_1 (Fig. 7.3)
Proceeding from superior to inferior, the deepest layer of the acetabular floor is formed first by the strong echoes of the inferior rim of the iliac bone; then by the echo-lucent triradiate cartilage; then by the strong echoes of the ischial bone. These are invested first by the echo-poor loose connective tissue of the acetabular fossa, which thus lies in front of the deep structures on the image, and superficial to this again by the ligament of the head of the femur. In this way a typical three-layered structure is formed, varying from above down in the composition of its deep layer.

Section b_1
A somewhat different echo pattern is produced along section b_1. The superficial layer of the echoes of the acetabular floor is still made up of the strong reflections from the iliac bone, but caudal to this is the whole of the descending limb of the triradiate cartilage. This limb is made of hyaline cartilage and gives rise to an echo gap that reaches far distally. Since the ultrasound beam is now not hindered by any bony structures, it passes through the descending limb of the triradiate cartilage and meets the perichondrium and the iliopsoas muscle within the pelvis on its inner side. Superficial to the triradiate cartilage lie the weak echoes

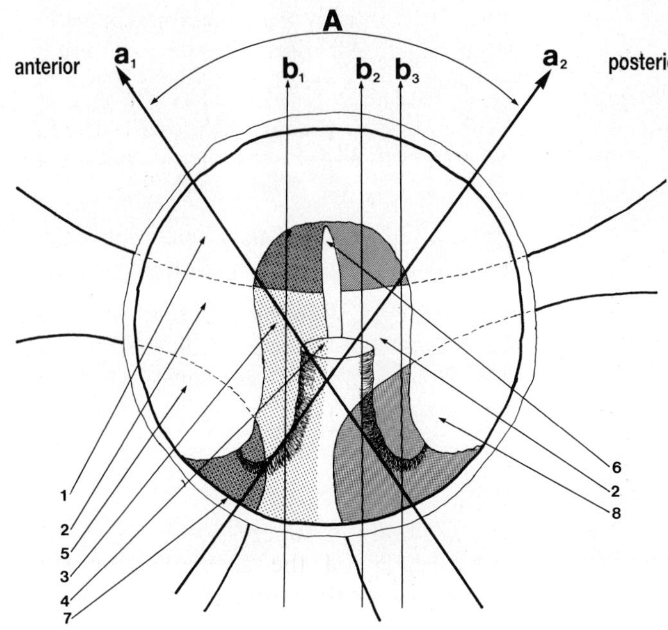

Fig. 7.2. Left hip. Schematic drawing of the left acetabulum corresponding to Figure 7.1.

a₁ This cut runs from anterosuperior to inferoposterior
b₁, b₂, b₃ Pure coronal cuts
a₂ This section runs from superoposterior to antero-inferior
1 Lunate facies
2 Horizontally running limb of the triradiate cartilage
3 Tissue of the acetabular fossa, partially dissected away
4 Ligament of the head of the femur
5 Pubic bone covered by the lunate fascia
6 Cut surface of the dissected tissue of the acetabular fossa
7 Transverse ligament of the acetabulum
8 Ischial bone

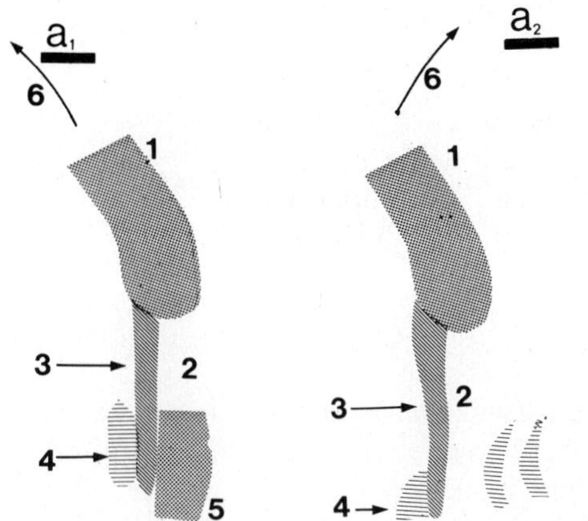

Fig. 7.3. Echo structure corresponding to the planes of section in Figure 7.2

a₁ and a₂ Rotated sections
b₁, b₂, b₃ Coronal sections
1 Os ilium
2 Echo poor zone of the hyaline triradiate cartilage
3 Tissue of the acetabular fossa
4 Ligament of the head of the femur
5 Ischial bone
6 Contour of the iliac bone

(The planes of section are directed forwards in a₁, backwards in a₂. In the planes of section b they run directly upwards.)

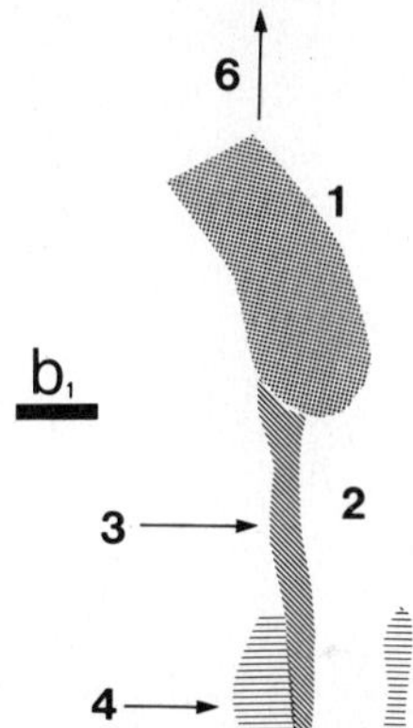

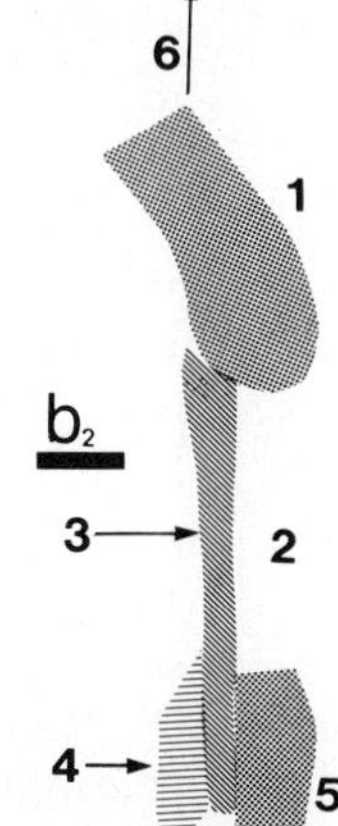

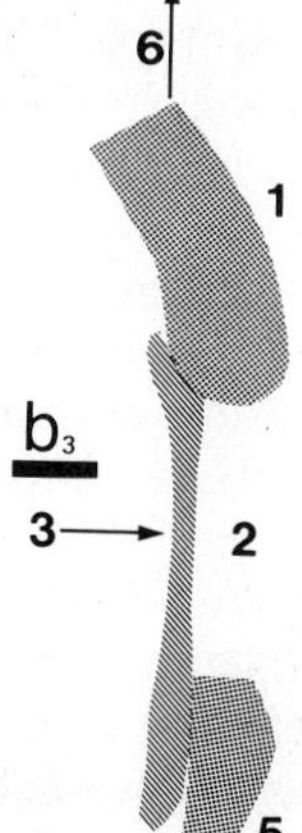

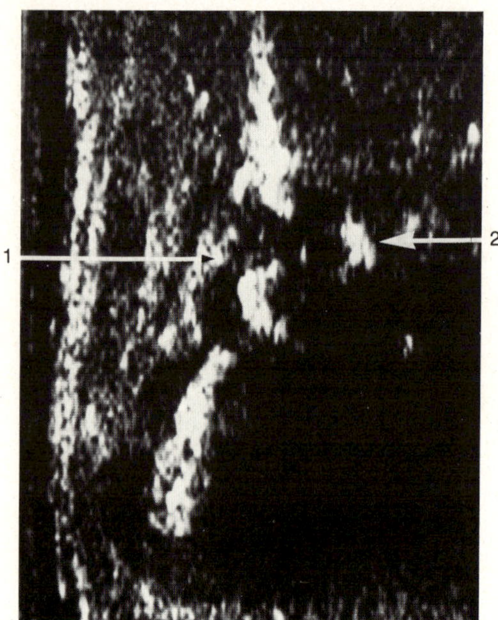

Fig. 7.4. Correct image section

1 Acetabular labrum
2 Iliac bone. The iliac bone with its inferior edge
   is seen clearly and distinctly

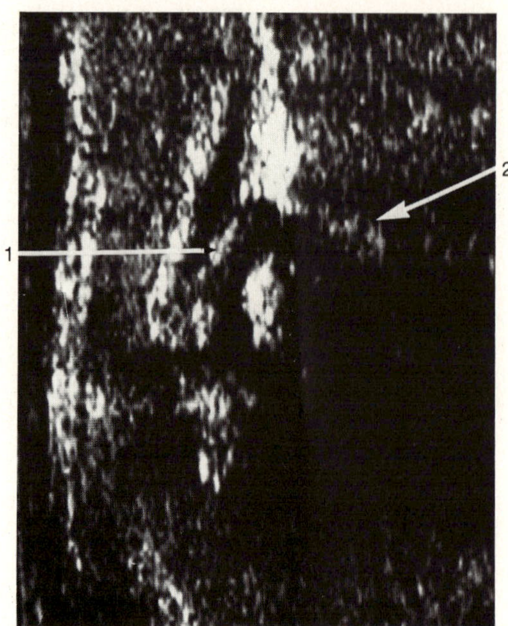

Fig. 7.5. Imaging section outwith the acetabular fossa. Key as in Figure 7.4. The inferior edge of the iliac bone is not seen clearly or distinctly but 'flutters' away towards the medial edge. This cut cannot be evaluated

formed by the loose connective tissue and, superficial to this again, the strong echo of the ligament of the head of the femur.

Familiarity with these anatomical details is necessary if the examiner is to orientate himself within the acetabular fossa.

However if section a_1 is compared with section b_2, it can be seen that these sections lie close together in their caudal parts and cannot be differentiated by their echo structures in the acetabular fossa. These cuts cannot be put in order solely on the strength of the different echoes of the acetabular fossa. Moreover, when the femoral capital ossification centre becomes large, the structures of the caudal part of the acetabular fossa fall into its acoustic shadow and are hidden. In contrast, the lower border of the iliac bone, being the furthest cranial structure of the acetabular fossa, remains visible even when the capital epiphysis is large. This lower border in the acetabular fossa thus forms the first vital landmark towards allowing a

reproducible and assessable section to be obtained (compare Figs. 7.4, 7.5).

7.2.2 The contour of the iliac wing

The varying contours of the iliac bone cranial to the acetabular rim can be utilised to define a section which shows the inferior border of the iliac bone more exactly and thus further defines a section within sector A in Fig. 7.3. The outer cortex of the ilium above the acetabular roof is doubly bowed, convex in a horizontal direction and with a concavity in the coronal plane increasing from before backwards (Fig. 7.1). On section a_1, with the probe rotated far anteriorly, the iliac wing sweeps out laterally above the roof of the acetabulum. When the plane of section is rotated towards the true coronal position (b_1 or b_3), then the contour of the ilium cranial to the acetabulum takes on an increasingly straight course running directly

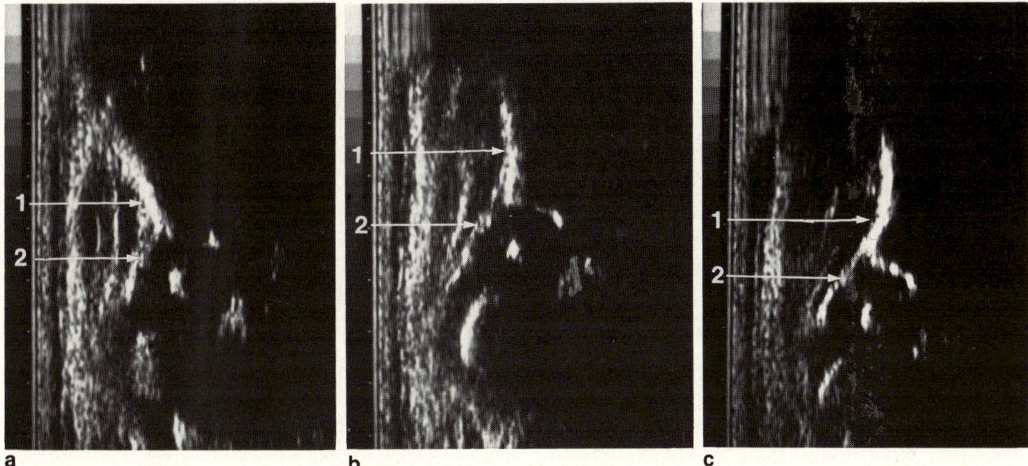

Fig. 7.6a–c. Three cuts taken at different places through the same hip joint

1 Contour of iliac bone
2 Acetabular labrum

a The line of this cut passes through the front part of the acetabular roof and the contour of the iliac bone rises laterally. The bony formation appears deficient. The cartilaginous part of the acetabular roof is widened.

b Correct plane of section. The contour of the iliac wing runs straight upwards.

c This section runs over the hinder part of the edge of the acetabular roof into the gluteal fossa. Correspondingly, the contour of the iliac bone is concave and arches medially. The promontory of the rear part of the acetabulum corresponding to this is rounded into a hump

upwards. Even further posteriorly, in the direction of the plane of section a_2, running dorsally over the back edge of the acetabulum where it forms a bony hump, the iliac wing falls sharply away and takes on a concave form through the trough of the gluteal fossa. With the help of this knowledge, the area of the acetabular roof can be scrutinised from ventral to dorsal and back, and thus an over-view of the whole load-bearing part of the acetabular roof can be obtained.

Practice has shown that it is unimportant whether the coronal section through the acetabular fossa is taken through the front part (cut b_1) or the rear part (cut b_3). However, as a standardised section for measurement, only the middle or true coronal cut should be taken (see § 7.1.1 above) (Fig. 7.6).

7.2.3 The acetabular labrum

This forms the third indispensable landmark for definition of the standard plane. Its prin-

cipal anatomical relationships are given in § 5.9, together with the most reliable procedure for identifying it (the 'standard situation').

7.3 Definition of the standard plane

A sonographic section can be used for assessment when and only when the following image criteria have been fulfilled:

1. Demonstration of the inferior border of the iliac bone.

2. Correct placing of the section over the area of the acetabular roof.

3. Demonstration of the acetabular labrum.

Practical procedure for obtaining the desired section is dealt with in chapter 12.

The only exception occurs in dislocated joints in which the femoral head is luxated craniodorsally and has migrated out of the standard plane, leaving the inferior border of the iliac bone behind. In this situation one generally has to leave the standard plane in order to demonstrate the dislocated femoral head in its relationship to the deformed cartilaginous acetabular roof. In these cases a measurement is not necessary anyway since dislocated (Type III and Type IV) hips are not distinguished from each other by measurement but only morphologically taking into account the direction of the deformation of the acetabular roof.

If the baby is kept horizontal and on its side then the contour of the ilium is generally parallel to the lateral edge of the image. This is a practical coincidence but can in no way be taken as a definition of the standard section. First, because the silhouette of the ilium may in fact be bent due to the individual form of the acetabular roof. Secondly, subluxed hips produce a naturally oblique plane but may simulate an anterior section through a healthy hip so closely that the silhouette of the section alone cannot be applied for differentiation.

In Fig. 6.2d to f and Fig. 6.13 the precision of the sections is demonstrated. Although in the radiograph (Fig. 6.2e) the development of the socket appears correct at first sight, sonographically a type II is present (Fig. 6.2d). This corresponds to a severe disturbance of ossification in the whole of the weight bearing area of the acetabular rim (marked with arrows in Fig. 6.2e).

7.4 Measurement techniques and mistakes of measurement

7.4.1 Introduction (Fig. 7.7a, 7.7b)

Measurement lines in radiographs can usually be made between clearly-defined points. In contrast, the end-points of measurement lines in sonograms are much less mathematically exact and more ill-defined, and adaptation of such lines for use on sono-

grams can only be done with qualified exactitude (Niethard & Roessler 1987). Experience has shown that mistakes are made over and over again in the construction of the sonographic measurement lines. In the following section therefore we will deal in more detail with the techniques and mistakes of measurement.

The measurement system proposed is artificial in that the measurement lines can be constructed upon the sonogram perfectly well but cannot be translated into histological sections. It is only one of 24 systems we have tested, and although it is not perfect, it is superior to all others in daily practice. Attempts to measure further angles arising from the bony angle α and the cartilaginous angle β have not improved the accuracy of the basic system. The advantage of the angle measurement systems lies in that the proportions of the acetabular roof and the relationship between the bony and cartilaginous parts of the roof remain unchanged regardless of the size of the hip that is being measured. This fact, and the consequent avoidance of unnecessary errors in measurement, can considerably raise the precision of the measurement technique, so that the range of error does not exceed 4°.

7.4.2 The acetabular roof line
(Figures 7.8a, b, 7.9, 7.10)

The point of origin of the acetabular roof line is the inferior point of the iliac bone in the acetabular fossa. The line is constructed laterally from here tangential to the bony echo (Figure 7.8a). This definition holds good both for sharp bony rims and for rounded or flattened ones.

Errors usually arise because of difficulty in localising the lowermost point of the iliac bone on the sonogram. The ilium in the acetabulum lies sheathed in connective tissue and overlaid by the ligament of the head of the femur and echoes from either of these may be confused with the ilium. The following methods may be used to identify the ilium (Fig. 7.8a):

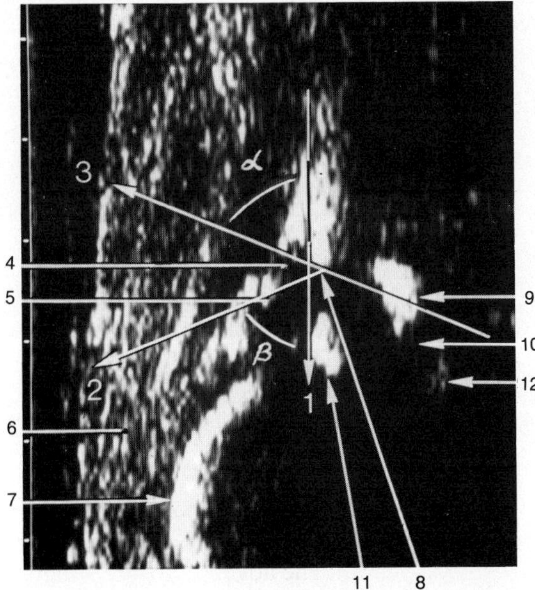

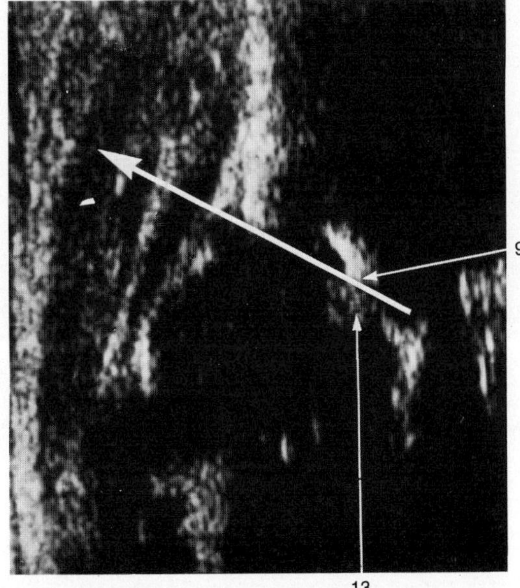

Fig. 7.7a. Measurement lines.

1 Baseline
2 Cartilaginous roof line
3 Acetabular roof line
4 Cartilaginous promontory
5 Labrum
6 Greater trochanter
7 Osteochondral junction
8 Bony promontory
9 Iliac bone
10 Triradiate carilage
11 Femoral capital epiphysis
12 Ischial bone
α Bony angle
β Cartilaginous angle

Fig. 7.7b. Precise localisation of the inferior border of the iliac bone facilitates a clear distinction between this and the tissue of the acetabular fossa. Compare 7.7a. Same key as in Figure 7.7a.

13 Tissue of the acetabular fossa

1. If the ultrasound machine is *not correctly adjusted*, the echo of the iliac bone may appear to be elongated caudally by the echoes of the connective tissue.

2. The bony ilium gives a *stronger echo* than that of the soft fatty tissue of the acetabular fossa.

3. The tissue of the acetabular fossa lies laterally (in front of) the lower border of the ilium on the sonogram. Caudal to the bony echo of the iliac bone is the echo-poor zone of the hyaline triradiate cartilage. Thus, the echo stripe of the connective tissue appears to be constricted from behind below the ilium by the echo gap of the cartilage: the so-called *tailoring* of the shadow.

4. Instruments with particularly high resolution may be able to differentiate three different *forms of the iliac bone* (Graf and Schuler 1986) (Fig. 7.8b):
a) The classical form,
b) The goblet-shaped form,
c) The 'frayed' shape.

A useful trigonometrical method is to locate the tip of the iliac bone, place the point of a pen upon it, and rotate a ruler around the point until it lies just tangential to the underside of the bony roof before drawing in the line.

7.4.3 The base line (Figs. 7.11–7.13)

The base line (erroneously also known as the 'iliac wall line') runs along the lamellar bone of the iliac wing and through the base of the cartilaginous part of the roof. It origin-

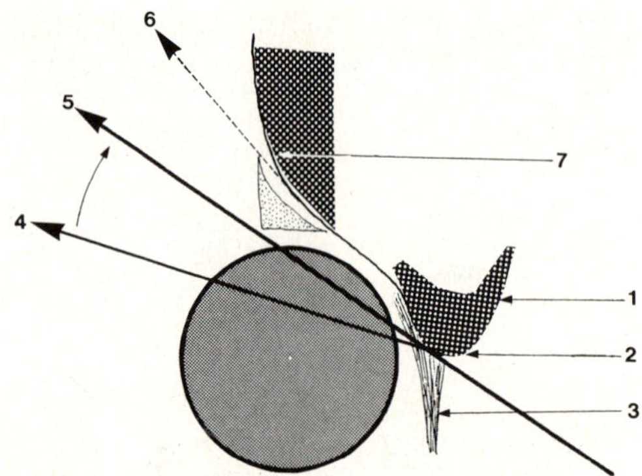

Fig. 7.8a. Scheme for the construction of the acetabular roof lines, in the case of an angular promontory (5) and of a rounded one (7).

1 Iliac bone
2 'Tailoring'
3 Tissue of the acetabular fossa

The line of the acetabular roof is lain tangential to the bony promontory. It is turned from 4 to 5 (in the case of an angled promontory) and to 6 in the case of a rounded one

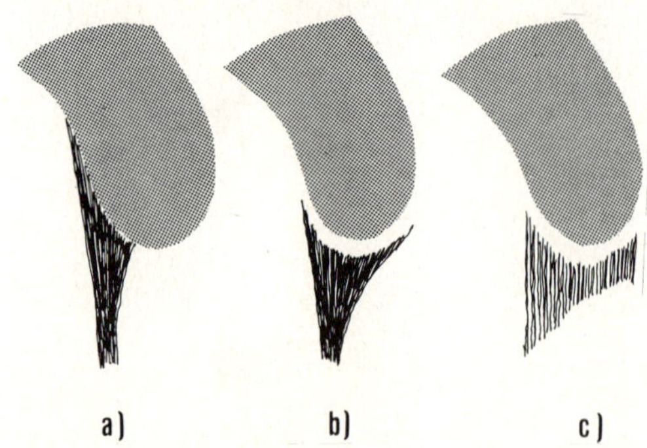

Fig. 7.8b. Sonographic forms of the inferior border of the iliac bone

a) Classical form
b) Cut form
c) The „frayed" type

ates from the most proximal (superior) point of the cartilage of the acetabular roof, where the periosteum lies in contact with the perichondrium and the ilium, and is constructed tangentially along the echo of the iliac bone (Fig. 7.11). This definition of the base line, as with the acetabular roof line, remains valid both for sharp bony rims as well as for rounded or flattened ones.

The contact point 'Z' is the junction between endochondral and periosteal growth (Oelkers 1981). Errors have been caused when the measurement line has been drawn from a point cranial to the true junctional point (point Z in Fig. 7.11), and this should be avoided. The length of bone upon which the base line can be drawn is extremely short even when it is taken from the true point Z, so if a sonogram is not available with the minimum magnification of 1:1, it is almost impossible to draw in the base line with adequate precision. It is thus mandatory to produce sonograms as large and as exact as possible so that accurate measurements can be made.

Once this superior point of the base line has been identified, a similar method is helpful as with the construction of the base line: place the tip of a pen upon the point and then rotate the ruler around it until the ruler lies just tangential to the iliac wall. This usually gives an accurate position along which to draw the line.

This proximal fixed point 'Z' cannot always be clearly identified, as the junction between the structures may either be over-insonated due to maladjustment of the machine, or it may be concealed by secondary ossification. This problem can be solved like this: an ultrasound beam approaching from the side is evenly quenched by the lamellar bone and medial to it an acoustic shadow is formed, in which the border between the echo-bright and echo-poor zones appears to represent the inner border of the cortex of the bone. This is an artefact and does not represent the true inner cortex, but it does lie parallel to the outer cortex and thus to the original base line. This line along the border of the acoustic shadow is known as the *accessory line*. Either the base line or the accessory line along the back of the acoustic shadow can be used to measure the bony angle, depending upon

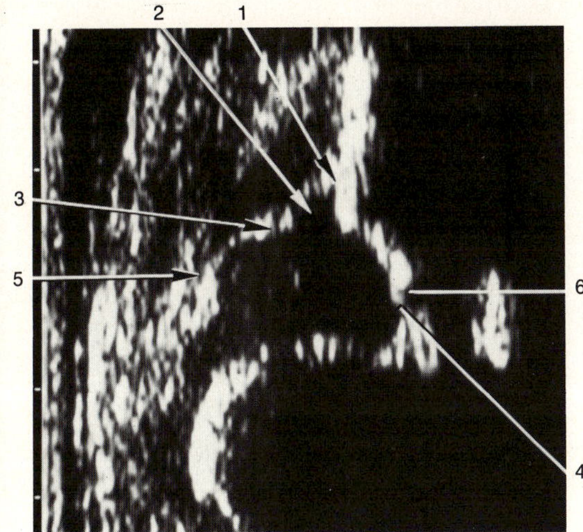

Fig. 7.9. The tissue of the acetabular fossa forms the tip of the echo and makes the echo of the iliac bone appear elongated.

1 Apposition of cartilage to bone
2 Cartilaginous acetabular roof
3 Acetabular labrum
4 Tissue of the acetabular fossa (the 'echo tip')
5 Joint capsule
6 Inferior border of the iliac bone

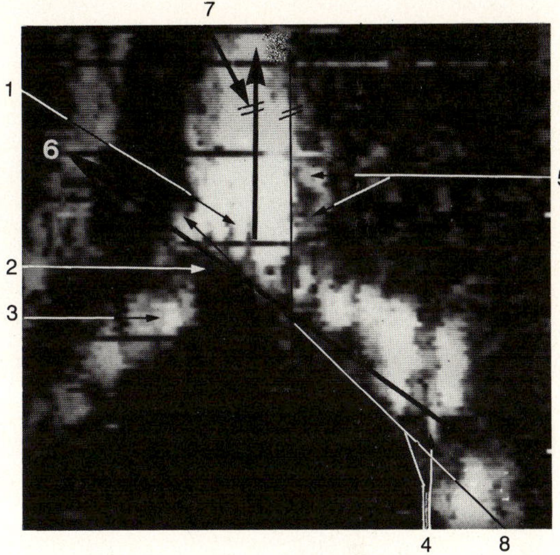

Fig. 7.10. Enlargement of the area of the acetabular roof with an acetabular roofline constructed tangentially and the tissue of the acetabular fossa

1 Apposition between cartilage and bone
2 Cartilaginous acetabular roof
3 Acetabular labrum
4 Tissue of the acetabular fossa
5 Scattered echoes
6 Acetabular roofline
7 Baseline with an accessory line through the back of the echo shadow.
8 Wrongly constructed acetabular roof line

which of them can be constructed with the greater precision.

The bony angle α, used as a measure of the development of the bony socket, is found between the base line and the acetabular roof line.

The base line is found on sonograms only and cannot be transferred a priori to histological sections.

7.4.4 The cartilaginous roof line

The line of projection of the cartilaginous part of the roof is the line that connects the bony rim to the acetabular labrum. It forms the angle β with the base line, and measures the degree of projection of the cartilaginous part of the roof.

The bony rim

Identification of the bony rim can cause difficulty in those cases in which the contour of the acetabular roof takes a curved or bent course. The question then arises of where the 'corner' lies on a curve. For this purpose, the point of the bony rim is defined as the most infero-lateral part of the bony acetabular roof, and is located at the point where the bony contour undergoes transition from concavity to convexity. In rounded or flattened bony rims, the transitional point can be defined exactly enough as the most inferolateral point on the acoustic shadow in the acetabulum (Fig. 7.14). It is also the point at which the acetabular roof line touches the roof.

In practice one should localise the bony rim by starting at the concavity of the acetabular socket, i.e., the bony rim is approached from the depths of the acetabulum, working towards the echoes of the lamellar bone. If

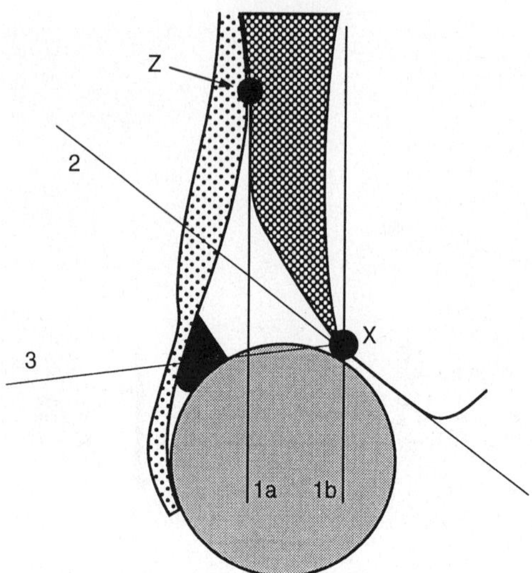

Fig. 7.11. Schematic measurement lines. The baseline is constructed from point Z tangentially to the bony echo of the iliac bone (1a). This runs parallel to the accessory line (1b) drawn down the back of the acoustic shadow thrown by the iliac wing. The acetabular roof line is drawn from the inferior tip of the iliac bone tangential to the acetabular roof (2), and the cartilaginous roof line (3) runs from the transitional point (X), where the curve of the acetabular roof changes from convex to concave, through the middle of the echo of the labrum

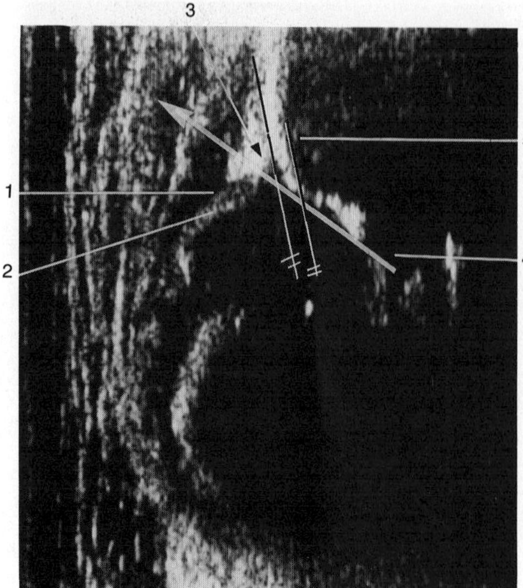

Fig. 7.12. Sonogram with baseline and acetabular roof line. The baseline (5) lies parallel to the accessory line through the back of the echo shadow.

1 Perichondral echo gap
2 Labrum
3 Secondary ossification
4 Acetabular roof line
5 Baseline and accessory line

one proceeds in the opposite (craniocaudal) direction, the rim is generally erroneously identified as lying too far cranially.

The acetabular labrum
To be anatomically correct, the measurement line should be drawn through the tip of the labrum. This can however not always be demonstrated, as it often lies closely applied to the joint capsule and exceeds the resolving power of the equipment. So the line is drawn through the main echo of the labrum (Fig. 7.15).

Note that the point of intersection of the base line and the acetabular roof line is not always at the bony rim. This intersection only happens to overlie the point of the bony rim only in type I hips with sharp and well-contoured bony rims.

7.5 Comparison of ultrasound techniques

As the interest has increased in sonographic examination of the hip, other imaging planes of the hip joint have been tried out (Clarke et al, 1985, Harcke et al, 1984a, Morin et al, 1985, Teot et al, 1988). A review of these possibilities had already been published by Graf (1980).

7.5.1 Advantages of the frontal approach

Any disturbances of maturity of the hip are found in the acetabular roof. So with a coronal plane of examination the whole of the acetabular roof can be examined in one

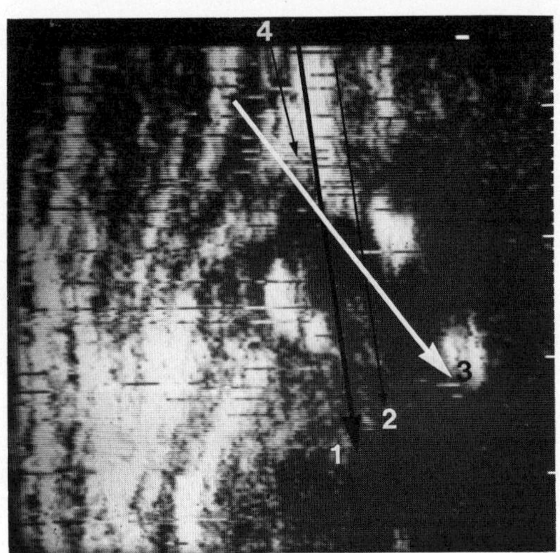

Fig. 7.13. Measurement error in the baseline in a case of secondary ossification.

1 Baseline correctly indicated
2 Accessory line through the back of the line of extinction of echoes
3 (White line) falsely constructed baseline. This line certainly touches the bony promontory but the proximal fixed point has been laid wrongly in the zone of secondary ossification (4)

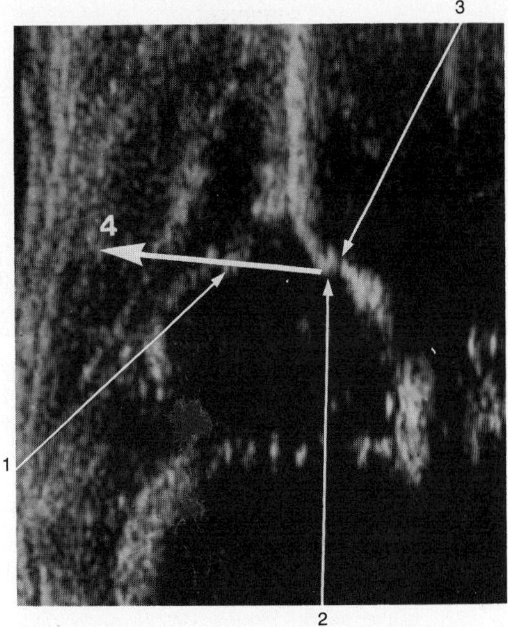

Fig. 7.15. Demonstration of the transition point for construction of the cartilage roof line.

1 Acetabular labrum
2 Transitional point
3 Acoustic shadow at the transitional point
4 Cartilage roof line

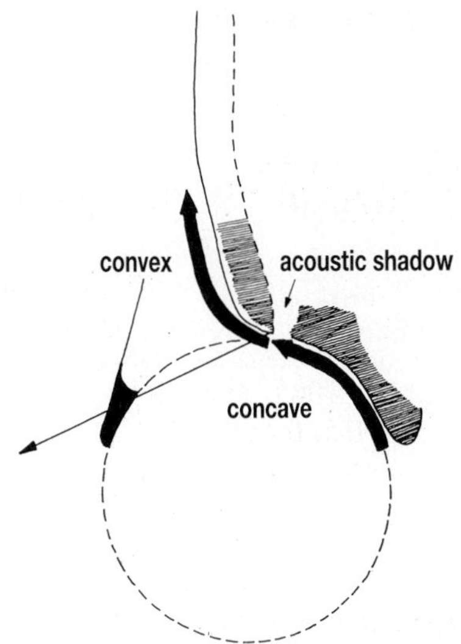

Fig. 7.14. Schematic drawing for the location of the measurement point for the cartilaginous roof line. This point is formed by the transition from concavity to convexity in the acetabular roof and is marked by an acoustic shadow which is more or less pronounced

tomogram, and the bony and cartilaginous relationships of the acetabular roof can be exactly classified. The femoral head luxates in a craniodorsal direction, so the coronal plane of section also makes it possible to form an objectively measured definition of instability.

In a consensus conference (Graf, Harke, Clarke, 1993), a minimal standard examination was established:

1. Imaging of a coronal standard plane with measurements and quantification, and

2. A dynamic stress test.

7.5.2 The 'internal approach'

This was described by Teot et al (1988). The infant is lain on his back and the femora are abducted. The ultrasound beam is then directed in a ventrodorsal direction into the groin. Thus the ultrasound beam meets the most ventral and the most dorsal parts of the acetabular roof but not the craniolateral edge. With this direction of insonation the placing of the femoral head in the socket may be checked. Instability is visible but is difficult to quantify as suitable parameters are not available. Detailed diagnosis of the acetabular roof cannot be carried out as the ultrasound beam does not strike those cranial and craniodorsal parts of the acetabulum which are relevant for estimating dysplasia. The anatomical orientation is relatively difficult. The examination itself provokes the infant to restlessness and crying as abduction with an instability test following upon it is less well tolerated than with a coronal direction of insonation with the infant positioned on its side.

7.5.3 The transverse approach

First described by Suzuki, this involves laying the infant on his back and placing a long ultrasound transducer against the front of the infant. It is used to visualise both hip joints together by directing the beam towards the posterior. As with the internal approach, detailed diagnosis of the acetabular roof is not possible as only the ventral and posterior parts of the acetabular roof can be demonstrated.

7.5.4 Posterior approach

If the infant is turned on to its stomach and the hip joint is examined by insonation from behind, then a luxation of the femoral head dorsally into the gluteal fossa can be made visible. This plane of insonation however only enables complete subluxations to be discovered, without any subclassification. We have not used this method since 1980.

7.5.5 The Lorenz position

It is quite possible to use an ultrasound plane through the adductor compartment with the leg abducted (the Lorenz position). Images taken of the femoral neck in the Lorenz position using a ventrodorsal direction of the beam enable one to make a sonographic measurement of the degree of antetorsion of the femoral neck (Dorn et al 1986). It is indeed possible to use this direction of cut to assess the correct position of the femoral head after reduction of dislocated hip joints but there are unavoidable technical difficulties in this type of examination and the results are difficult to quantify. This technique is not routinely used and does not produce any additional information (Clarke et al 1985, Graf 1980, Novik et al 1983, Teot et al 1988).

7.5.6 The Harcke technique

Harcke also uses the lateral approach, but tests only the stability of the joint using the so-called dynamic or stress examination. See 'consensus conference' above. Instability is not quantified and is not distinguished from physiological movements. No account is taken of the fact that a stable joint is not always normal and healthy.

Key points

- A standard measurement plane needs to be defined in order to carry out reproducible measurements of the acetabular roof.

- The cardinal landmarks used to define the standard plane are:
  The lowermost edge of the iliac bone,
  That section through the iliac wing which shows it rising vertically away from the acetabulum,
  The acetabular labrum.

- In dislocated joints, the femoral head may lie outside the standard plane.

- The principal measurement lines are:
  The acetabular roof line, drawn from the iliac tip along the bony echo of the acetabular roof,
  The base line, drawn along the bony echo of the iliac wing,
  The cartilaginous roof line, drawn from the tip of the labrum to the infero-lateral extremity of the bony rim.

- The principal angles for measurement are:
  The bony angle α, measured between the bony roof line and the base line,
  The cartilaginous angle β, measured between the cartilaginous roof line and the base line.

8 Determination of hip maturity with the sonometer

8.1 The sonometer

We have investigated the detailed anatomy of the infant hip by performing arthrograms on hip joints and comparing them with sonograms prepared at the same time. We took into account the age of the patients as well as the bony and cartilaginous relationships of the acetabula, paying meticulous attention to the projections. These bony and cartilaginous relationships can be expressed as angles, the α and β values, which could be arranged together by comparison of the radiological findings in each age group with the corresponding sonograms. This naturally showed that high α values represent good bony roofing, usually with correspondingly small cartilaginous parts manifested as a relatively low β value. However, as will be discussed later, high β values may also be found with well developed bony acetabula (§ 8.2). As the bony socket deteriorates, the α value diminishes. In consequence, with the compensatory increase of the cartilaginous acetabular roof, the β value rises. The nomographic arrangement of α and β values are known as a *sonometer* (Fig. 8.1).

If the α and β values are marked for each hip joint on the sonometer and connected by a straight line, an optical impression of the bony and cartilaginous development of the socket can be obtained. Three major divisions arise from this, readable from the sonometer:

(a) on the right hand side of the sonometer are the mature hips known as type I. In our present state of knowledge when the α *angle is 60° or greater*, the socket is developed to

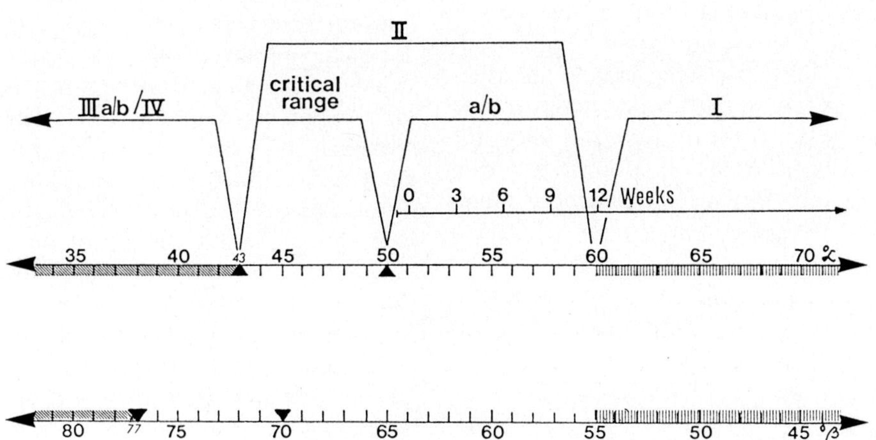

Fig. 8.1. Sonometer. Linear arrangement of α and β angles dividing up the types of hip (the β scale runs from right to left). On the right are the type I hips and on the left the dislocated hip types IIIa/b and IV. In the middle lie the type II hips with the subdivisions into type IIa, IIb and also IIc. Time scale for newborn babies: the zero point at full term lies opposite 50° to 51° on the α scale. Twelve week limit lies opposite $\alpha = 60°$

such an extent due to the formative stimulus of the femoral head that no deterioration of the roof covering is to be expected with increasing age. (The only exception from this rule is well-known and occurs when the neuromuscular balance has been disturbed. So, for example in spastic diplegia, the disturbed biomechanics can lead to deterioration and eventually to subluxation.)

(b) at the left hand end of the sonometer stand the dislocated hips (*types IIIa and b and type IV*).

(c) *Type II hips* belong to the central region. This includes the various grades of severity of delay of ossification.

By arranging these types and angles, and by paying careful attention to examination technique, the exact position of the maturity of the hip from dislocated through to completely mature hips can be represented graphically.

8.1.1 Historical note

The arrangement of the angular parameters as originally tabulated in 1981 (Fig. 8.2) produced too rigid a division into types and nowadays must be considered to have been superseded, particularly as regards the β values, and in this form should be seen as of historic interest only. According to this scheme the hip joints were divided up into three categories. This however does not allow for the many possibilities of variation found in nature in the bony and cartilaginous development of the acetabular roof.

	α	β
Type I	60° and greater	55° and less
Type II	43° to 60°	55° to 77°
Type III/IV	43° and less	77° and greater

Fig. 8.2. Table of angles for the body angle α and the cartilaginous angle β arranged according to individual hip types. This table represents the state of knowledge in 1981 and is of historical interest only

8.2 Using the α and β angles to subdivide hip types

(Table 8.1)

8.2.1 Types Ia and Ib

Statistical investigations have shown that the average α value in hip type I is 64.4°. The average β value is 67.4°. This would mean that a hip with an α of 60° has reached the absolutely necessary degree of bony maturity in order to be treated as matured. Our present day knowledge suggests that an α of 60° should be described as a 'borderline normal finding.'

Cartilaginous rims may show remarkable variety in their degree of distinction even among type I hips with a correct bony formation ($\alpha = 60°$ or greater). On the one side there are the widely overlapping "peaked" cartilaginous rims which are drawn downwards over the femoral head and give rise to small β angles. Type I joints ($\alpha = 60°$ and greater) with β values of 55° and lower are known as *type Ia hips*. The small β angle is an expression of the narrow cartilage of the acetabular roof, passing far laterally and caudally around it.

On the other hand there are shorter, wider cartilaginous rims sitting upon the femoral head which have higher β angles. Type I hip joints ($\alpha = 60°$ and greater) with β values greater than 55° are known as *type Ib hips*. In this hip type the β value can often encroach over the 77° border. This high β value with joints where α is over 60°, is simply an expression of a short acetabular cartilage sitting directly on top of the femoral head (Figs. 8.3 to 8.5, Table 8.1). (Note that type Ib was referred to in the older literature as the so-called 'transitional form'. This concept of a 'transitional form' should not be used any more nowadays as it is misleading).

According to our present day knowledge, both type Ia and type Ib are seen as being physiological variants of a mature hip. When plain radiographs are taken of these pelves, the bony relationships are completely cor-

Table 8.1. Overview of division into types with descriptive findings

Type	Bony formation	Bony rim	Cartilaginous rim	a	b	Clinical implications
Mature hips (any age) Ia	Good	Sharp	Easily covers the femoral head	>60°	<55°	No therapy
Ib	Good	Usually curved ('blunt')	Short, and covers the femoral head	>60°	>55°	
IIa Physiological delay in ossification						
IIa(+) Appropriate for age	Adequate	Rounded	Covers the femoral head	50°–59°	>55°	No therapy – follow-up
IIa(−) With delay in maturation (up to 3 months of age)	Deficient	Rounded	Covers the femoral head	50°-59°	>55°	Follow-up in borderline cases, more usually treatment in abduction harness
IIb 'real' delay in maturation	Deficient	Rounded	Covers the femoral head	50°-59°	>55°	Treatment in abduction harness
IIc At-risk or critical hips (any age)	Deficient	Rounded or flat	Still covers the femoral head	43°–49°	<77°	Immediate therapy with abduction harness (will deteriorate if untreated)
D Hips on the point of dislocation (any age)	Severely deficient	Rounded or flat	com-pressed	43°-49°	>77°	Immediate therapy, stable fixation necessary
Dislocated joints IIIa	Poor	Flat	Displaced upwards, no disturbance of structure	<43°	>77°	Immediate treatment. Referral to specialist, reduction
IIIb	Poor	Flat	Displaced upwards, with dis-turbance of structure			Good position of the femoral head deep in the acetabulum is necessary
IV	Poor	Flat	Forced caudally	<43°	>77°	Immediate treatment, admission to hospital, reduction

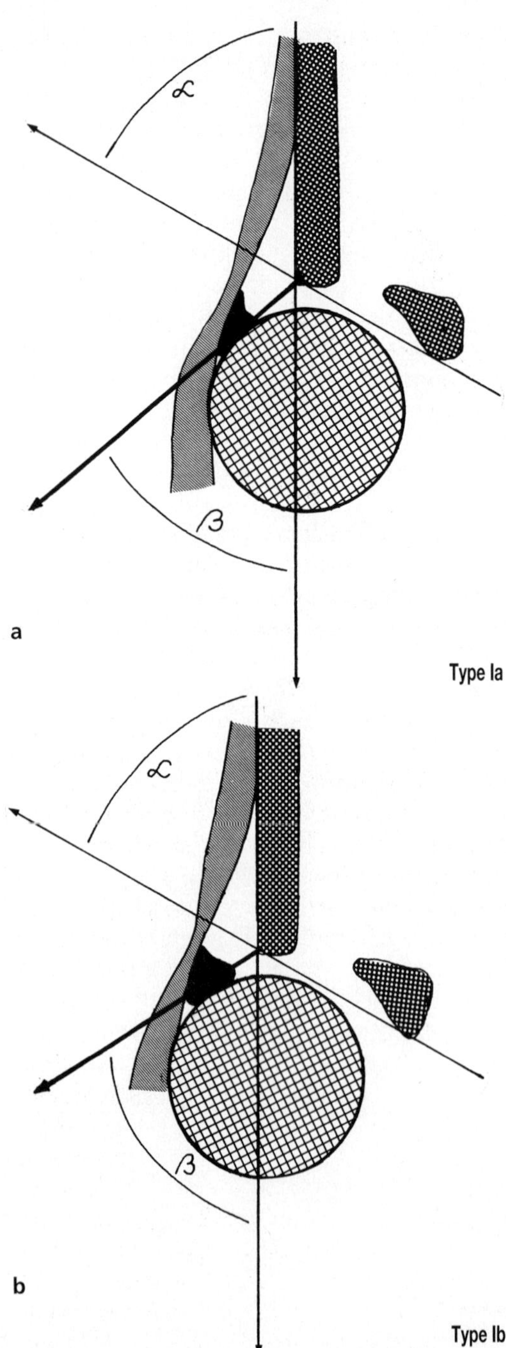

Fig. 8.3a, b. Schema for comparison of type Ia and type Ib hips. In both cases the bony rim is equally well developed. In Figure 8.3a α small β angle arises from the widely overlapping cartilaginous acetabular roof. The larger β angle (usually identified with a hip of at least grade II) shows there is a short wide cartilaginous acetabular roof sitting on top of the femoral head (Fig. 8.3b)

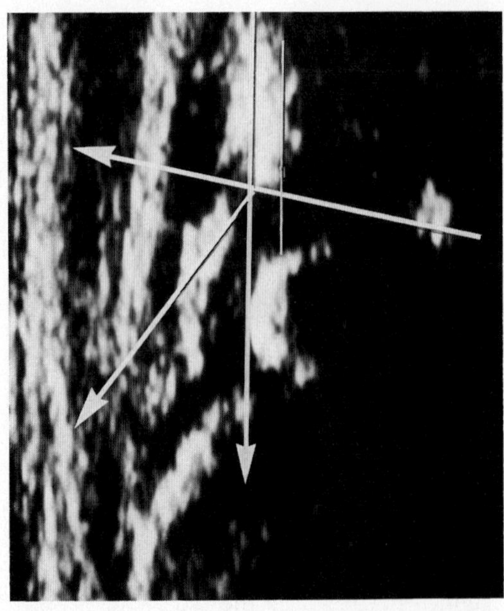

Fig. 8.4. 12 month old right hip joint. The measurement lines are drawn in. α = 78°, β = 37°. Hip type Ia (narrow, widely overlapping cartilaginous roof)

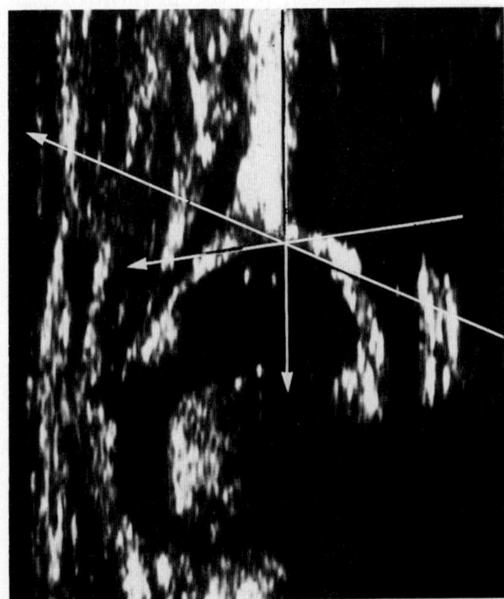

Fig. 8.5. Newborn hip joint. α = 66°, β = 80°. The cartilaginous roof sits on a broad base and overlaps the femoral head well. The base line is drawn in through the edge of the shadow deep to the iliac wing

rect and appropriate for the child's age. On the other hand such joints show variants of the cartilaginous acetabular roofs at arthrography corresponding to the ultrasound findings.

8.2.2 The causation of osteoarthrosis: a hypothesis

Naturally the cartilaginous rim starts to ossify after the end of the growth period, and thus type Ia and Ib hips give rise to differently shaped hip sockets in adulthood. On the one hand we find narrow acetabular roofs widely overlapping the femoral heads which arise from ossification of deep sockets. On the other side are the short cartilaginous roofs of the so-called 'small sockets', which never indeed fall into the true category of dysplasia. However, we believe that the variations in the biomechanics produced by either or both of these variations may give rise to pre-arthrotic deformities in later years. To date, these reflections are speculative and still await scientific proof.

This hypothesis does also not explain which hips the completely healthy ones are.

8.2.3 The newborn hip joint: hips type IIa, IIa(+) and IIa(−)

Newborn hip joints and joints up to the third month of life have to be allowed a certain degree of physiological delay in ossification. They may be deficiently formed in their bony formation in a physiological way and to a degree that depends upon the child's age. In general they show wide cartilaginous rims. These hips therefore should not be classed as showing 'delay in ossification', as this would lump them in with pathological hips. In order to take account of their unique situation, the term '*physiological delay in ossification*' is correct. We have typed these hips sonographically as *type IIa*, i.e., physiologically immature hips.

It has been shown that a newborn hip at birth should have reached a minimum degree of maturity ($\alpha = 50°$ to $51°$). On the sonometer the angle α of 50° to 51° stands opposite to the zero point (corresponding to a full-term delivery) on the timescale (Fig. 8.1). If the newborn hip has not reached this minimum degree of maturity then our experience shows that it will indubitably deteriorate and in the severe case can lead to subluxation.

Newborn hips which have reached this minimum initial degree of maturity should be expected to continue to mature steadily so that they reach normality (type I) by the third, or at latest the fourth, month of life. (This is shown on the sonometer, where the twelve week mark lies opposite the α value of 60°). If such hips are followed up sonographically at four week intervals, they should equal or exceed the minimum *acceptable linear maturation* in their α values corresponding to the timescale. These are *type IIa(+)* hips, normal for age, and under these conditions treatment is not necessary.

However hips that fail to keep up with this linear progression of maturation, but start to fall behind, should be treated at once, as if left untreated valuable time is lost and the hip may otherwise end up in the third month of life showing a manifest and true dysplastic delay in ossification. These are hip type IIa *with deficient maturation* – hip *type IIa(−)* (Table 8.1).

In the first six weeks of life it is difficult to take a measurement precise enough to make an exact differentiation between the various α values as during this whole time period of six weeks only 5° (between 50° and 55°) are available for assessment. Thus the sub-classification into IIa(+) and IIa(−) can in practice only be successfully used after the sixth week.

Hips which belong to type II and have the same α angles may have varying β values, analogous to the situation among type I hips. However, unlike type I hips, type II hips with the same α angles have a worsening outlook as the β angle rises. High β angles imply a short, squat cartilaginous rim, rather than a widely overlapping one, and this means that the total roof coverage will be poorer (Figs. 8.6, 8.7).

8.2.4 Delay in ossification after the third month (type IIb)

A hip which has fallen into the critical zone of the type II hips after the third month of life is known as a *type IIb* hip. For such hips the description of 'delay in ossification' is appropriate and corresponds radiologically to a dysplastic joint.

However, some scope for judgement is allowable in treating individual cases. If a baby reaches twelve weeks with a hip which is not yet quite mature, with an α value of just below normal, say 58°, then the transitional period can be carried over into the fourth month of life to allow for physiological maturation and normal variation. Such a hip may well mature spontaneously after a further four weeks and thus be spared treatment. On the other hand, if there is a considerable delay in maturation at the end of the third month of life, and particularly if there are also other negative factors such as a history of dysplasia in the family, a malposition in utero, breech presentation and so forth, then the safest path for the examiner to follow is to proceed to immediate therapy. This may then be broken off in four weeks at the next follow-up attendance if hip type I has been reached. Hips found to be type II after the fourth month of life are clearly dysplastic and should be treated without delay.

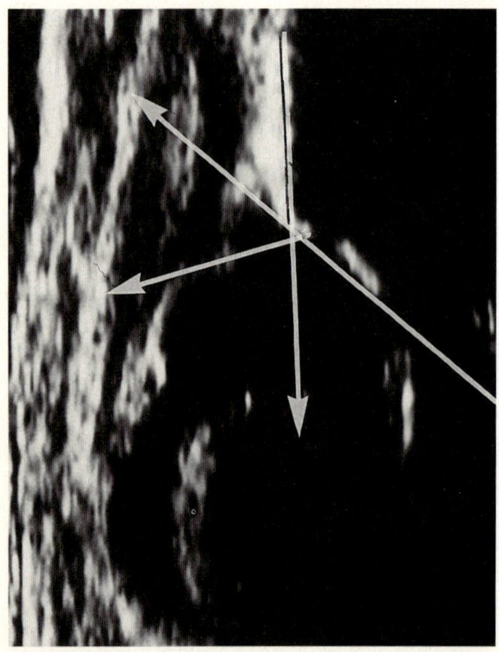

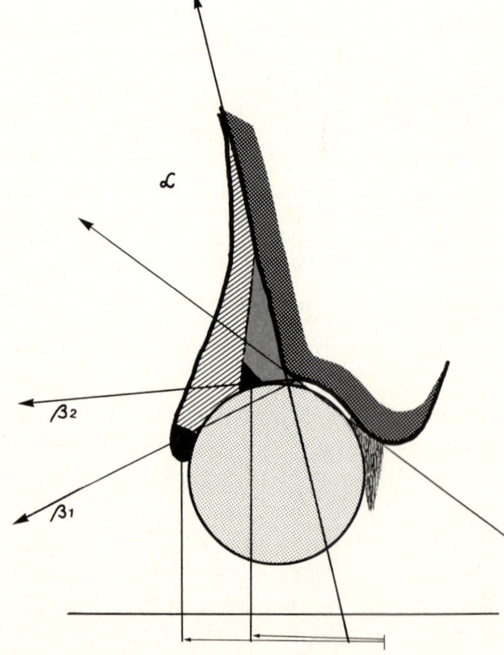

Fig. 8.6. Newborn hip joint. The bony formation is severely deficient, the bony rim is markedly rounded, the cartilaginous acetabular roof is wide but is however still overlapping the femoral head. α=48°, β=75°. Hip type IIg (=IIc)

Fig. 8.7. Relationships of the coverings of the acetabular roof. In the presence of equal α values, the hip with the small β value (β₁) is better covered than the one with the larger β value (β₂)

8.2.5 Classification of premature infants

In premature infants a certain degree of delay in ossification should be tolerated (Dorn et al 1987). Such hips are typed according to their calendar age. Therapeutic implications however are decided according to the gestational age. So for example, a four month old child born six weeks prematurely would be classified as a type IIb hip in order to document the deficiency in maturation. However, in assessing him for therapy, his age would be corrected for gestation, and he would be considered to be two and a half months old. This would leave him 'normal for age' and not in immediate need of treatment. Short term follow up in order to document clearly the maturation of the joint would still be necessary.

8.2.6 The stability of hip joints: type IIc

Hips which have not reached the minimum value of maturity at birth but have fallen into the left hand half of the type II range are called '*critical range*' or *type IIc* hips. They have such bad bony formation and are so highly dysplastic that, in our experience, they will inevitably deteriorate if left untreated and there is a danger of dislocation. These hips should therefore be treated immediately regardless of the child's age (Fig. 8.6). The α values of these hips lie between 43° and 49°, with a b value of less than 77°. There is a continuous spectrum of change between type IIa and type IIb hips on the one side and type IIc hips on the other.

Type IIc joints are usually *sonographically unstable*. This means that under compression (the stress examination) it is possible to

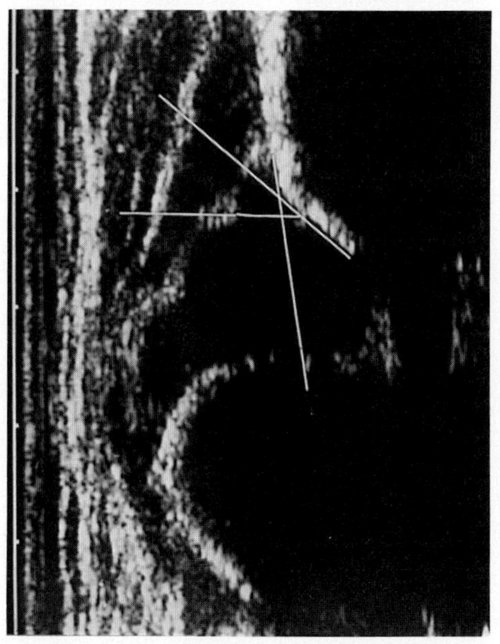

Fig. 8.8a. Four-week-old hip joint. The bony formation is severely deficient. The bony rim is markedly flattened. The cartilaginous acetabular roof is somewhat compressed cranially.

α = 45°, β = 105°. Hip type D

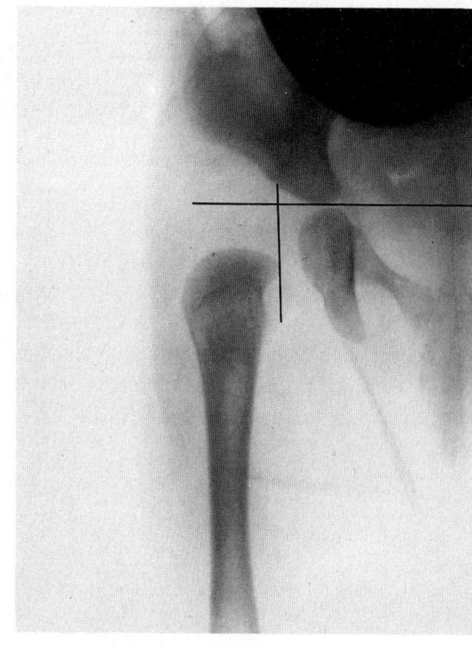

Fig. 8.8b. Radiograph to Figure 8.8a

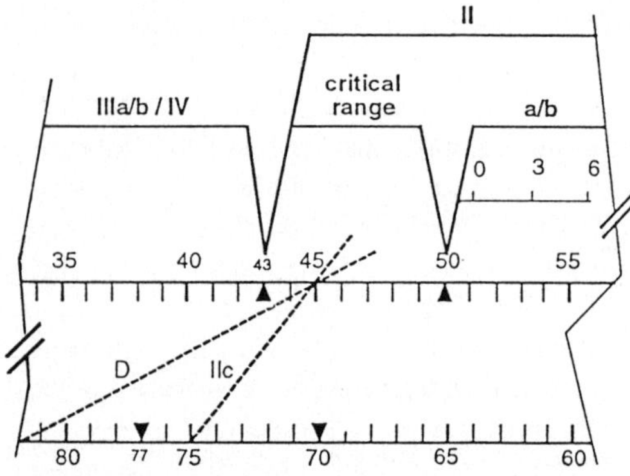

Fig. 8.8c. Differentiation between hip types IIc and D. In both types, α lies in the IIc range. In the type IIc hip, β<77°, in the type D hip β>77°

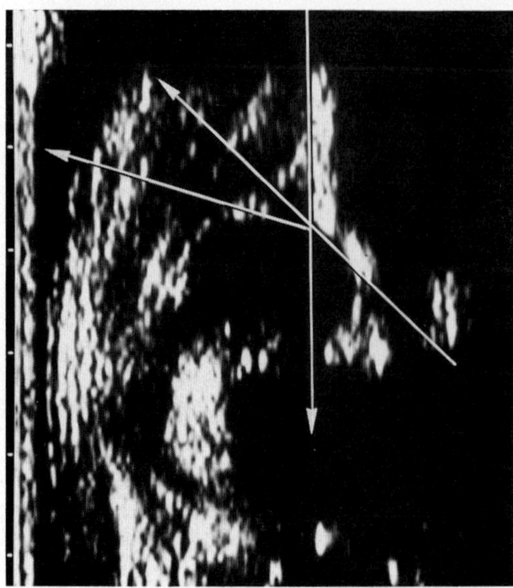

Fig. 8.9. Four week old hip joint. The bony formation is severely deficient, the bony rim is flat, the cartilaginous roof compressed. α=45°, β=105° hip type D

subluxate the femoral head out of the socket. This important procedure has received much attention in the academic press, and is dealt with separately in chapter 9.

8.2.7 Dislocated joints: types D, IIIa, IIIb and IV

Type D is the first stage of a dislocation. In these hips, the α value lies in the IIc range but the acetabular roof is deformed further upwards, and the β value rises above the cut-off point of 77° (Figs. 8.8, 8.9). This type should not be known as type 'IID', as a hallmark of all type II joints is that they are all centred in the acetabulum. Differentiation between type D and type IIIa is generally only possible by measurement technique: morphologically both types appear as dislocated.

The differences between hips of types IIIa, IIIb and IV were discussed in chapter 6. They are distinguished morphologically by the shape and texture of the acetabular roof cartilage, and not on the sonometer.

Key points

- The various combinations of α and β angles among hip types can be displayed graphically on the sonometer. In general, increasing levels of dysplasia are associated with falling α and rising β values.

- Among properly located joints only, the α angles are used for primary classification and the β angles for further sub-classification.

- Normal variation is allowable among type I hips (types Ia and Ib).

- Hips from the time of birth up to the third or month may mature spontaneously to some extent. They can be considered as maturing normally (type IIa(+)), failing to mature normally (type IIa(−)), or too dysplastic to be able to mature (type IIc).

- Hips which have failed to mature after the third month are called type IIb hips.

- Type IIc hips may divided into stable or unstable types on dynamic testing.

- Dislocated hips (types III and IV) are not distinguished by measuring angles on the sonometer.

With modern real-time equipment it is possible to demonstrate movements inside the body. By performing a dynamic examination, an examiner who also has responsibility for the patient's therapy can obtain a good overview of the relationships of the hip joint.

The baby is as usual laid in the lateral position. The transducer is placed in the normal manner and the hip is sonographically demonstrated. Now if the leg being examined is moved then the movement of the femoral head in the acetabulum can be followed.

9.1 Performing the dynamic examination

The practical conduct of the stress examination is shown in Fig. 9.1 (see also Chapter 12). After positioning the baby and application of the probe, the hip is examined in the normal way. The typing of hip joints is carried out in the position of rest, without stress. The probe is now kept exactly where it is, and the examiner with his other hand presses on the leg in a craniodorsal direction. Keeping the hip in slight adduction makes the instability if present more impressive. In sonographically unstable hips the femoral head rises taking the actebular labrum with it. When the compression is removed from the femoral head this springs back into its original position. In high grade defects of maturation the upward compression of the femoral head can be seen sonographically even when the baby spontaneously draws in its leg and the pull of the adductors compresses the femoral head upwards.

The essentially important phenomena to consider are the elastic suspension of the hip and signs of instability.

9.2 Natural elasticity of the hip joint

Even in completely mature hips a slight upwards flexibility of the acetabular labrum can just be seen when the proximal end of the femur is moved against the cartilaginous rim. It occurs because biomechanically and anatomically speaking the hip joint is ovoid and not completely spherical. This flexibility is an adaptation process and an expression of the physiological incongruence between the parts of the joint, which are compensated for by the accessory parts of the joint. This elastic suspension does not change the type to which the hip joint belongs, and of course the position of the femoral head can be judged both in adduction and slight abduction.

9.3 The unstable hip joint

Clinical testing of stability as a basic element of any clinical examination of the infant hip depends upon the anatomy of the hip, the experience of the examiner, and not least upon the muscle tone. Testing of instability would actually only be ideal if the muscle tone were abolished by anaesthesia. Otherwise an instability of the hip may be missed in a restless and possibly powerfully struggling infant.

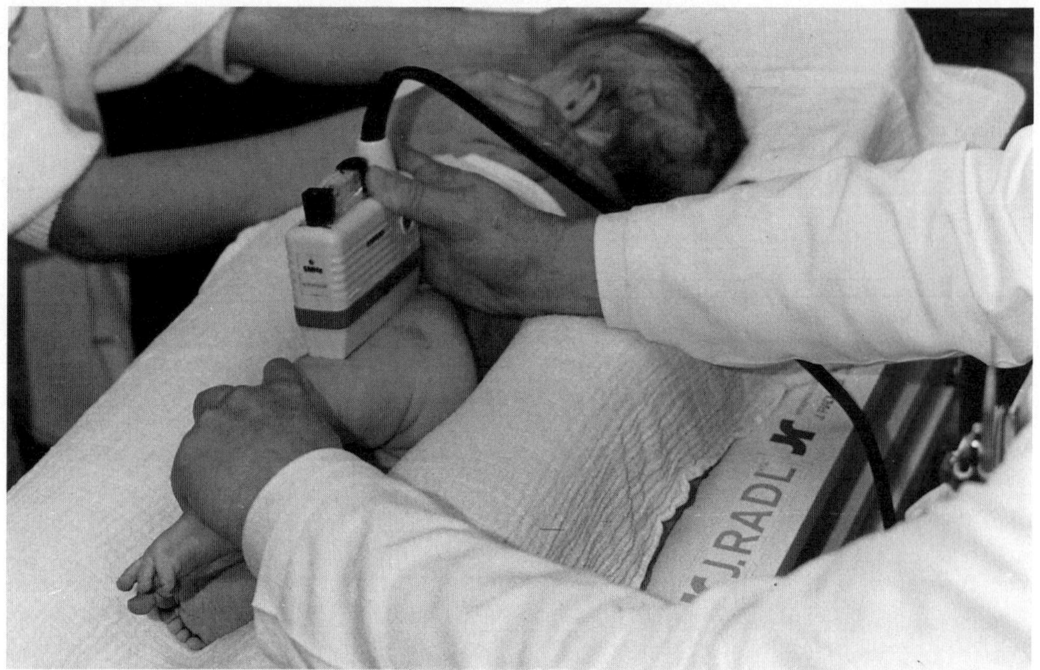

Fig. 9.1. Stress examination of the left hip joint. The right wrist rests on the cushion of the cradle, in order to allow the transducer to be handled securely. The left hand grasps the limb being examined and can apply compression and traction to the hip joint

Naturally dislocated hip joints are intrinsically unstable (Types D, IIIa, IIIb and IV). Among the less severely dysplastic hip joints, it becomes important to decide at what point a hip joint actually becomes unstable; how sharply can the border between stable and unstable hips be drawn?

This borderline is paramount, and subdivides the type IIc joints. *A hip joint starts to become unstable* sonographically if the β value rises over the defined value of 77° in a hip with an α value in the IIc region. When a stress test is applied to an unstable or type IIc hip, the cartilage of the acetabular roof is bent cranially and the femoral head becomes eccentric, and may raise the β angle above this value. This hip is known as a hip joint 'on the point of subluxation' or hip *type IIc unstable* or *type D* (Figs. 8.8 and 8.9). As nothing has changed within the bony part of the acetabular roof, the α value remains unaltered.

If a Type IIc hip cannot be dislocated under pressure, and the cartilaginous part of the acetabular roof cannot be bent beyond the defining measurement of $\beta = 77°$, then this hip joint is known as *Type IIc stable.*

Distinguishing between these two types enables the examiner to define the instability by measurement and objectively, and independently from subjective clinical impressions (Figs. 9.2a and 9.3a to c).

Hips with fixed dislocations may be further dislocated during a dynamic examination. Thus a type III hip with a high dislocation can be transformed into a type IV hip if the femoral head can be pushed further cranially, and the cartilaginous roof can be completely slid beneath the femoral head and squashed between the that and the iliac bone. Such a hip would be classified as type III rather than type IV because the basic typing of the hip is carried out in a position of rest.

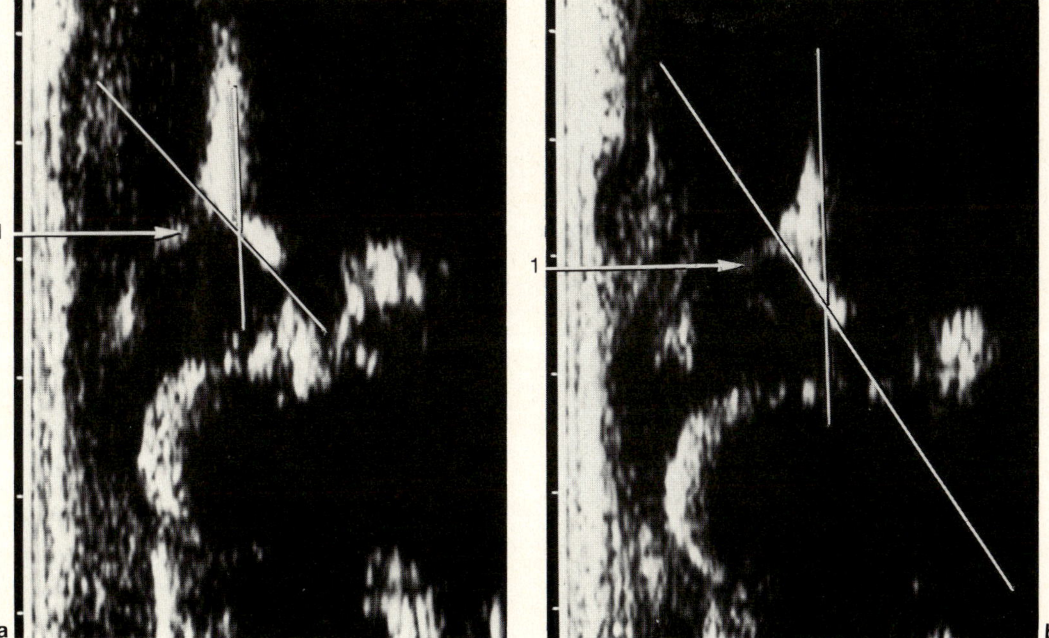

Fig. 9.2a, b. Sonographically unstable hip, 14 days old.

a Initial position. $\alpha = 45°$, $\beta = 90°$, hip type D.
b Under compression, the labrum is forced cranially. $\beta = 120°$. 1 = Labrum

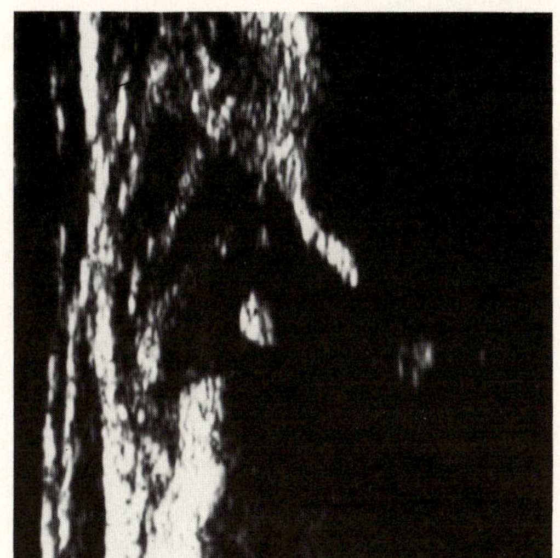

Fig. 9.3a. Initial position without compression or traction. The bony formation is bad, the bony rim flat, the cartilaginous roof is compressed upwards and is echo-poor. Type IIIa

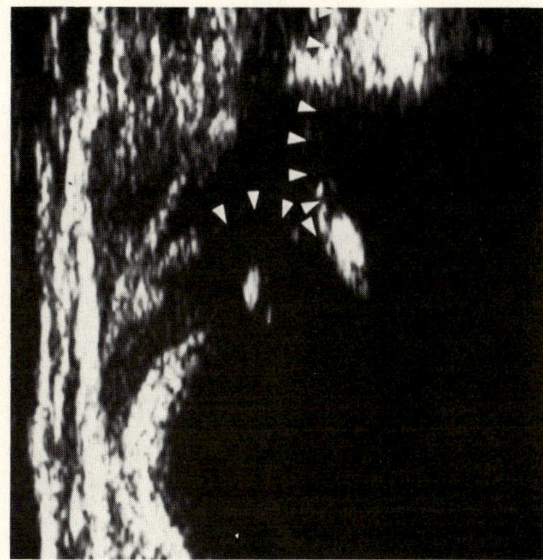

Fig. 9.3b. The same hip joint as in figure 9.3a under compression: the femoral head moves clearly further up, and has now left the true acetabulum and is dislocated cranio-dorsally. This cranio-dorsal situation of the femoral head is recognised by the posterior plane of the section

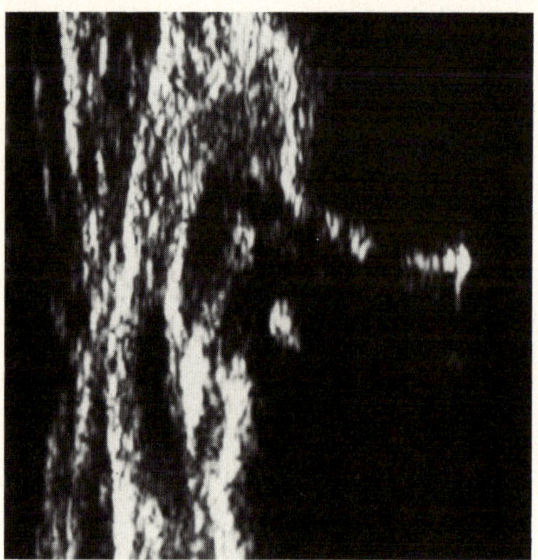

Fig. 9.3c. The same hip joint as above under traction. An attempt to relocate the hip results in the femoral head being well replaced in the true acetabulum. The labrum now covers it well

A differentiation must be made between clinically and sonographically unstable hips (see also chapter 13).

9.4 The Ortolani phenomenon

The Roser-Ortolani sign is a clicking sound that can be elicited in the first days and weeks of life in an unstable joint by lateralizing the femoral head by compression and adduction and then allowing it audibly and palpably by a process of separation of the thighs to spring back into the centre of the acetabulum. Understandably, the question arises of the sonographic equivalent of the Ortolani phenomenon. The anatomical bases of the Roser-Ortolani sign are described by Ortolani (1937, 1951, 1978), and Stanisavljevic (1964, 1982) and by Doerr (1968). Sectioned preparations in children with the Ortolani phenomenon showed considerable deformity of the cartilaginous acetabular rim in a dorsocranial direction caused by the femoral head compressing it from underneath. A tiny ledge forms itself at the junction between the already somewhat compressed limbus and the true acetabulum that Ortolani referred to as the *neolimbus*.

According to him the clicking sound is caused by the femoral head gliding to and fro over this neolimbus. According to Stanisavljevic the beginnings of such a secondary acetabulum are not always demonstrable. The Ortolani sign was investigated arthrographically by Tönnis, (1984), Schwetick, (1976) and Peic (1975).

9.4.1 Tönnis's definition of the Ortolani sign

Tönnis pointed out the distinction between the Roser-Ortolani sign and other tests of dislocation of the hip such as the Barlow test. According to Tönnis, in the Roser-Ortolani test the femoral head jumps back into the acetabulum because of the elasticity of the capsule and its bindings. It may also be displaced by compression and adduction. In the Barlow test the femoral head remains in a luxated position.

In cases with a clinical Ortolani sign we can establish the following by sonographic investigation:

1. Every single case shows a hip with a high grade deficient bony formation and a wide cartilaginous rim. These are the hips which the sonometer shows to be either in the critical zone, 'on the point of dislocation', or mild type III hips.

2. When these hips are examined dynamically, that is when pressure is exerted from caudal to cranial, they become definitely worse. The femoral head is pressed upwards out of its original place, taking the cartilaginous acetabular roof with it. This sonographic instability can also be shown in severely immature hips in the critical zone without a definitely demonstrable Ortolani sign.

It is thus mandatory to carry out and document a sonographic check on the stability in all hips that belong to Type IIc or worse.

See § 13.3 for remarks concerning the implications and safety of the Ortolani phenomenon.

Key points

- The stress or dynamic examination is performed by applying compression along the length of the femur.

- The natural elastic properties of the joint should not be mistaken for instability.

- Many type IIc joints dislocate (or become unstable) when the dynamic test is applied, and the β angle then rises to over 77°.

- Hips showing a positive Ortolani sign have a deformed roof with a secondary ridge or neolimbus.

- Some sonographically unstable hips are Ortolani negative, so dynamic testing should be carried out on all type IIc hips.

10 Reporting the hip sonogram

10.1 Components of the sonogram report

It is absolutely necessary to use unified terminology in the description of the sonographic findings of the hip joint. An exact report must include the following points:

1. The age of the patient
2. A description of the findings
3. The α and β angles
4. The hip type
5. Therapeutic implications

10.1.1 Age of the patient

The age must be given because it restricts the number of hip types to be considered. For example, a four month old hip cannot be classified as a Type IIa – type IIa refers to a physiologically immature hip under the third month of life only. The natural tendency of the hip to mature should be assessed in the light of the child's age.

10.1.2 Description of the findings

The bony and cartilaginous relationships of the acetabular roof should be described separately. Definite sonographic terms have been adopted so that if the cartilaginous and bony parts of the acetabular roof are correctly described, then this necessarily leads on to the correct hip type.

For better diagnosis and to facilitate subclassification, the bony rim (the 'contour of the rim') and the formation of the bony socket (the 'bony formation') should also be explicitly distinguished, as they do not necessarily go hand in hand with each other. It is true that a sharply contoured bony rim is usually associated with good formation of the socket, giving a high bony angle and good bone formation. However in an extreme case, a poor bony formation can be seen, with a low bony angle α and a radiologically shallow acetabulum. When this begins to heal, the rim may become sharp as a sign of increasing improvement of the relationships with the acetabulum, although the socket itself is still shallow. The improving contour of the rim recognisable at an early stage is a prognostically favourable sign even when the bony formation itself is still deficient.

The cartilaginous acetabular roof is described according to its formation and its sonographic structure. The concepts of bony formation, bony rim and the description of the cartilaginous rim are seen in Table 10.1.

10.1.3 Further definitions

Type Ib hips. In hip Type I one does not always find the classically sharply contoured, angulated rim. Instead of this the bony rim is often definitely rounded – the type Ib hip. We call this form of rim 'bent', 'blunt', or 'minimally rounded'. This matters because a bony rim which is in itself well contoured should be present caudal to the minimal rounding. If there is minimal rounding of the well contoured bony rim, then there may be a thicker layer of cartilage which shows itself in a higher β value.

Abnormalities associated with dislocation. The concept of 'compression' of the roof cartilage automatically implies a dislocated hip. On the other hand, the concept of

Table 10.1. Description of findings: The concepts are assigned to specific types and are not transferable. The one exception to this is the descriptions of the type II hip. Here, as well as the usual descriptors 'adequate', 'deficient', and 'overlapping' (or 'covering the femoral head'), the word 'sharp' may be used to describe the start of secondary ossification in the acetabulum

Type	Bony formation	Bony rim	Cartilaginous rim
Mature hips (any age)			
Ia	Good	Sharp	(widely) overlapping
Ib	Good	Usually curved ('blunt')	(narrowly) overlapping
IIa			
Physiological delay in ossification			
IIa(+)	Adequate	Rounded	Overlapping
Appropriate for age			
IIa(−)	Deficient	Rounded	Overlapping
With delay in maturation (up to 3 months of age)			
IIb	Deficient	Rounded	Overlapping
'real' delay in maturation			
IIc	deficient	Rounded or flat	Still overlapping
At-risk or critical hips (any age)			
D	Severely deficient	Rounded or flat	Slightly displaced
Hips on the point of dislocation (any age)			
Dislocated joints			
IIIa	Poor	Flat	Displaced upwards, no disturbance of structure
IIIb	Poor	Flat	Displaced upwards, with disturbance of structure
IV	Poor	Flat	Diplaced caudally

'overlapping' or 'grasping' of the cartilage over the femoral head is reserved exclusively for centred hips. Meticulous use of these few concepts can help to avoid wrong diagnoses. For example it is contradictory to describe the bony formation as 'good,' the rim as 'angulated' and 'pronounced', and yet simultaneously to classify the acetabular roof as 'wide and compressed.' If indeed such phrases have been combined, they may give a first indication that a wrong diagnosis has been made.

10.1.4 Report on the angles

Construction of the measurement lines and calculation of the bony and cartilaginous angles are not principally done in order to arrive at a diagnosis; a practised examiner will do that from the monitor. However, the angles do confirm the diagnosis and make possible subclassification of the status of maturity of the hip joints. It follows that any report of the hip sonogram containing only the angles but without a textual description is not enough. The angles can be used as a cross-check upon the validity of the textual description, as can the compatibility of the various descriptive terms discussed above; they also have the advantage of being more objective than the textual description. Any inconsistency should prompt the examiner to double-check his findings.

Key points

- Consistency of reporting of the hip sonogram demands that a strictly defined set of terms should be used.

- Any inconsistency within the report should be checked, as it may indicate an error in interpretation of the images.

11 Positioning and manual technique

11.1 General conduct of the examination

One problem of the sonographic examination of the joint is that of obtaining exactly the correct plane of section each time. This involves structures whose lengths are measured only in millimetres; and on top of this the infant is often moving itself. In order to facilate this even for unpractised examiners, standardised techniques for positioning and palpation have been developed which can be learned and practised. In this way the best hip sonogram can be produced in the shortest possible time.

We always conduct the *sonographic examination first*, and only add the clinical examination afterwards. If the reverse order is followed then one has to deal with a considerable unrest and irritation in the infant during the sonographic examination due to the clinical examination already carried out.

As has been discussed in the previous chapters, the system for judging the infant hips on the sonogram is independent of the baby's posture, making it in principle irrelevant how the baby is positioned. However, we have found it best to *lay the baby on his side* and direct the ultrasound beam in the coronal plane so that the greater trochanter forms the point of contact against the transducer. The baby should be as comfortable as possible in the side position into which he is placed and should have warm and soft coverings. In this way it can be assured that he lies as calmly as possible during the process of the examination.

11.2 The cradle apparatus and positioning

We have constructed and tested in practice for many years a positioning apparatus which functions like a hammock with an elastic fastening[1]. It consists of two softly upholstered pads with somewhat larger hollows for the torso and pelvis than for the legs (Fig. 11.1a–d). A napkin or diaper is laid loosely over the pads which is held down on the outer sides either with 'Velcro' or by a rubber band. The infant is then laid upon the hammock formed by this napkin. The examiner can make the hollow deeper or shallower according to the size of the infant, so that the hip to be examined remains lying a little proud of the side pads. All other apparatuses for fixing the baby in a restricted position during the examination have shown themselves to be unsuitable and we have abandoned them.

It is convenient to carry out the examination in the standing rather than the seated position. A small table or cot should be provided, suitable to the height of the examiner, on which the positioning apparatus can be lain or fastened. This enables the examiner readily to examine the baby from the side. He can support his forearms comfortably on the edge of the table and control the ultrasound transducer without difficulty. Care must be taken all the same that neither the examiner nor the mother, if she is assisting, should pull on the baby's legs, as this leads to a slight outward rotation of the hip. Fixing the hip in this position

---

[1] Manufacturer: Fa. Radl KG, Luthergasse 4, A-8010 Graz, Austria. Patent applied for.
Agent in Germany: Fa. Popp GmbH, Geuderstrasse 11, D-90489 Nürnberg, Germany

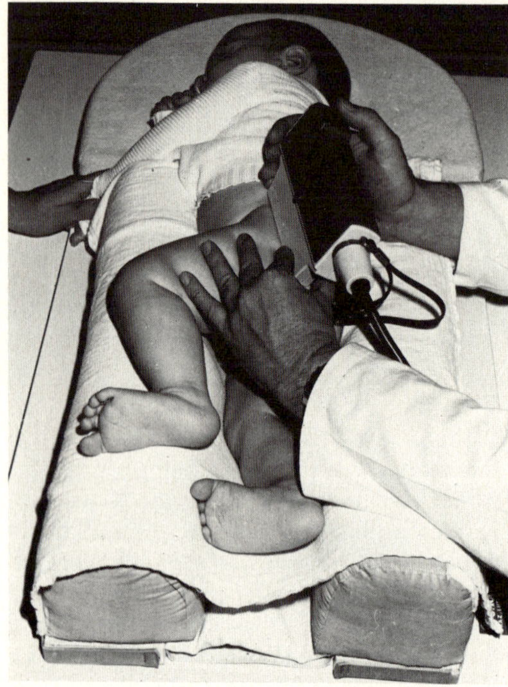

Fig. 11.1a. Incorrect positioning and palpation technique. The leg has slid forwards over the side pad of the cradle. The greater trochanter is rotated somewhat dorsally making the palpation technique more difficult

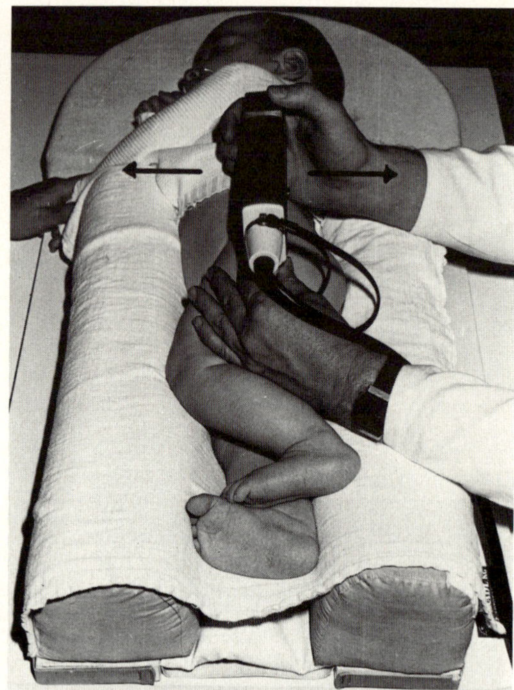

Fig. 11.1b. Correct positioning and palpation technique. The leg is slightly inwardly rotated and the knee has not slid out over the side pad. The initial position is shown with the transducer positioned perpendicular to all the spatial planes. The arrows demonstrate the "search path"

upsets the infant and it also slides the ultrasound probe dorsally or ventrally off the contact point on the greater trochanter. As a rule it is much more appropriate to keep the position taken up spontaneously by the infant.

The natural position of the hips in slight flexion does not disturb the conduct of the examination. A slight inward rotation draws the greater trochanter from dorsal to ventral so that the greater trochanter, the neck of the femur and the acetabulum lie on the same coronal plane. This favourable inward rotation can be accentuated if the examiner presses the knee joint downwards with his wrist within the support. On no account should the knee project out over the side pad because this will make the greater trochanter rotate dorsally. This makes the technique considerably more difficult.

Figure 11.1a shows a wrong position for comparison with the correct positions in Fig. 11.1b to d.

11.3 Finger and hand position (Fig. 11.1a to d)

Production of a correct hip sonogram should in no way be left to chance. We recommend that a systematic procedure be followed:

In recent years we have realised that the transducer and the baby must be handled very precisely. The right hand, generally the more skilled side, has the main work in the management of the transducer, and the left hand is predominantly involved in fixation of the child. If the *right hip joint* is being examined, the left middle and forefingers

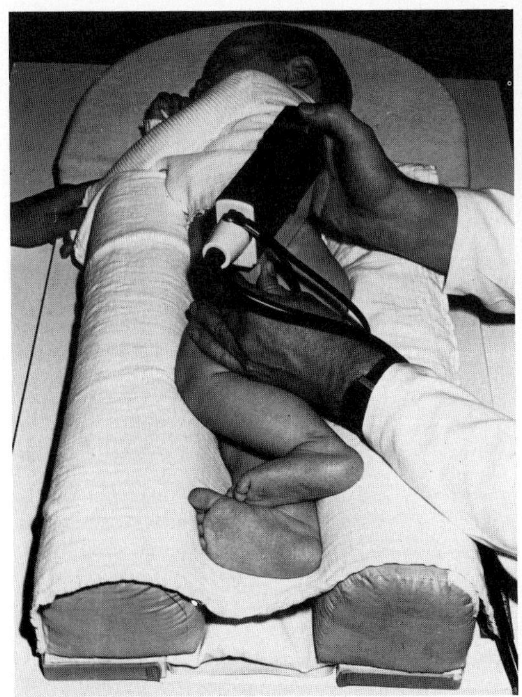

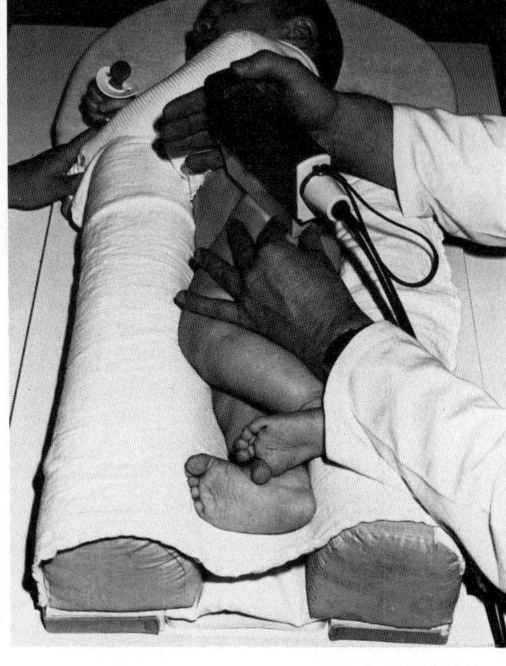

Fig. 11.1c. Section over the posterior edge of the acetabulum

Fig. 11.1d. Section over the front edge of the acetabulum

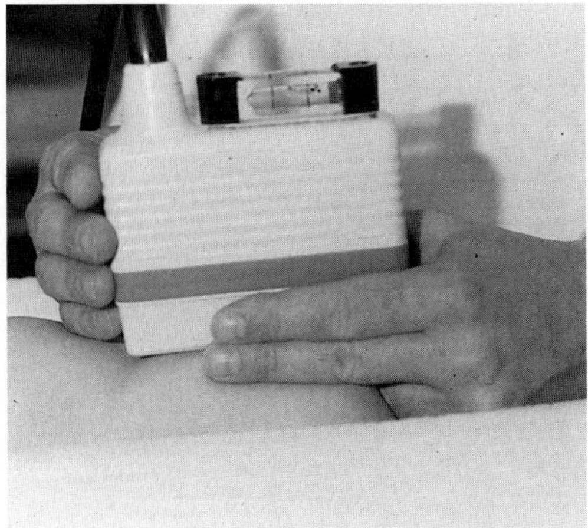

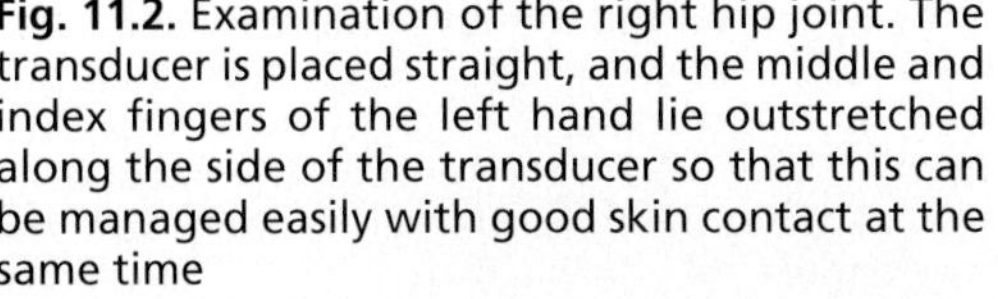

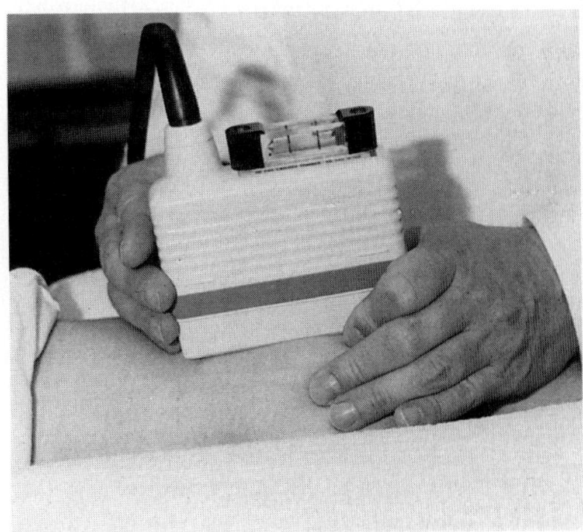

Fig. 11.2. Examination of the right hip joint. The transducer is placed straight, and the middle and index fingers of the left hand lie outstretched along the side of the transducer so that this can be managed easily with good skin contact at the same time

Fig. 11.3. Incorrect finger position. The infant may be irritated by the pressure of the pads of the fingers and apart from this the transducer cannot be directed confidently over the greater trochanter with the infant restless

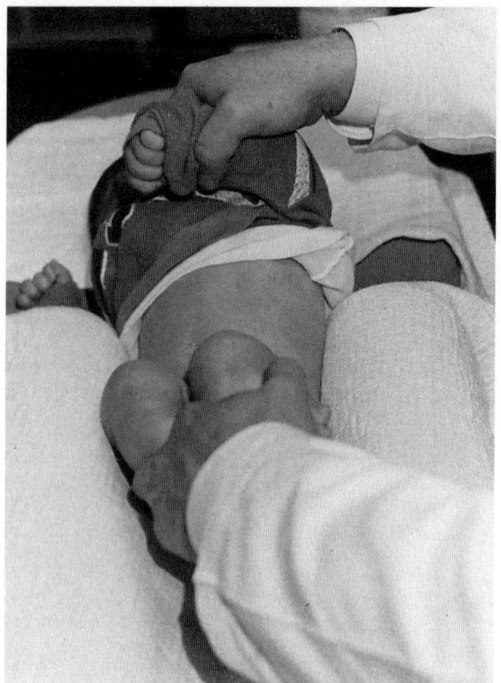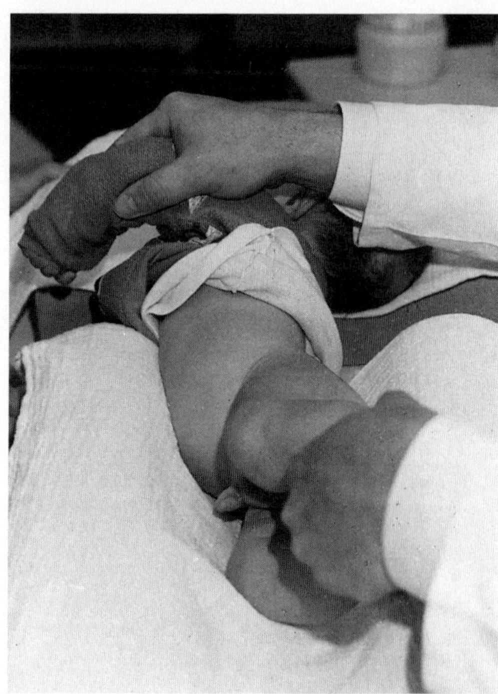

Figs. 11.4 and 11.5. Procedure for turning the baby. The examiner's left hand grasps the infant's leg. The infant's left arm is then gently raised and the baby is turned without drawing it out of the cradle

should be laid outstretched along the back side of the transducer so that good management of the transducer can be obtained at the same time that contact against the skin is maintained (Fig. 11.2). Since both forearms are supported comfortably against the side pads of the cradle, the transducer can be reliably managed even when the infant is restless. Under no circumstances should the middle and index fingers be bent as the pressure of the balls of the fingers can irritate the child and provoke unrest (Fig. 11.3).

Turning the child over from the right to the left hand side should not be left for the mother to do. The left hand of the examiner grips the infant's ankle, while the right hand lifts the child by drawing lightly on the left arm and turns it over on to the other side with a simultaneous rotation movement without lifting it significantly out of the cradle (Figs. 11.4 and 11.5).

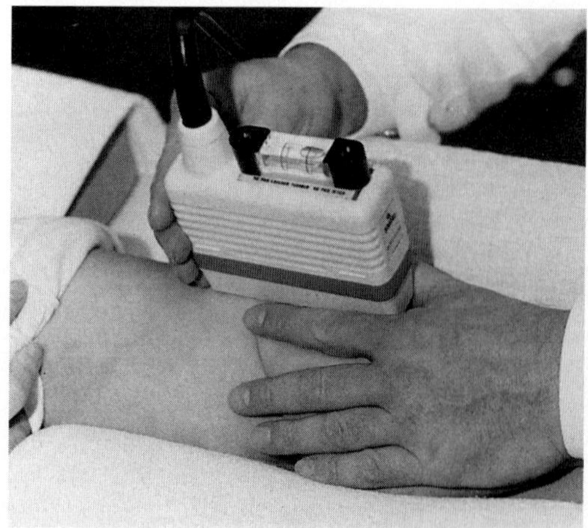

Fig. 11.6. Examination of the left hip joint. The left hand is laid flat so that the outstretched fingers surround the infant's thigh and push the knee joint downwards at the same time. The thumb and index finger surround the transducer so that the greater trochanter lies between the two fingers

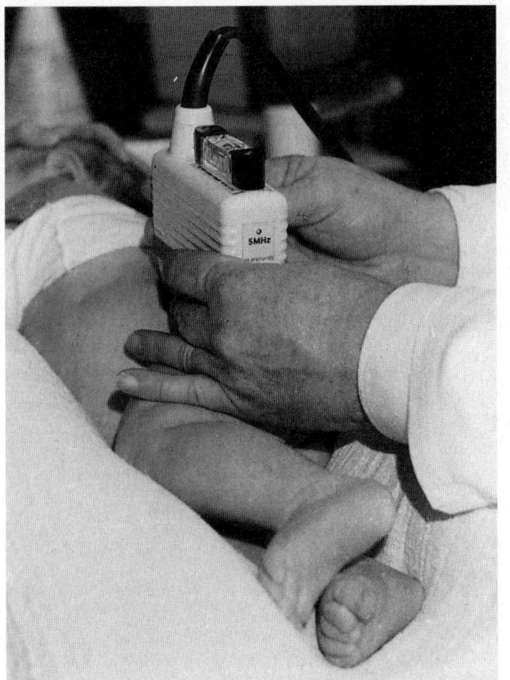

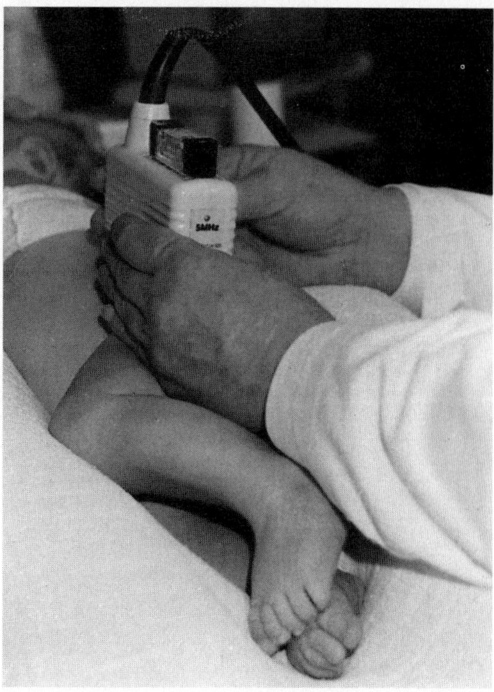

Fig. 11.7. Incorrect hand position. When the child is restless, the examiner may reflexly push it downwards. The child may be irritated by the pressure of the side of the hand

Fig. 11.8. Incorrect hand position. As in Figure 11.7 this restless baby cannot be examined because the hand has not been laid flat and because the thigh and shin have not been adequately fixed. The infant's leg can slip out of the cradle

During the examination of the *left hip joint* the examiner's left hand is laid flat against the infant's leg. This also has the effect of fixing the infant's leg with the knee bent (Fig. 11.6). With the flat of the examiner's hand this can be fixed even when the infant is restless without provoking the child to more distress by pressure from the edge of the hand (Fig. 11.7 and 11.8). The examiner takes the child from the mother. The mother assists and lays her hand on the baby's shoulder. The probe should be placed on the infant's hip perpendicular to all the spatial planes: it should lie exactly along the long axis of the infant without any angulation (Fig. 11.1b).

11.4 Manipulating the probe

In general the standard plane of section is hit upon immediately if the baby is in the correct position. If this does not happen immediately then a systematic search should begin in two main directions:

1. Sliding the probe. Hold the probe vertically without tipping it and gently slide it back and forth, keeping it parallel to the coronal plane, until the femoral head and the acetabulum are demonstrated. The main aim of this 'search path' is to find the joint, rather than to reproduce the precise standard plane of section within it. The inferior tip of the iliac bone is located by 'fine tuning' (small alterations to the transducer position). The picture is frozen as soon as the inferior border of the iliac bone is clearly visible.

Table 11.1

	Procedure	Comments
1	Take the child from the mother.	Mother to assist and lay her hand on the baby's shoulder.
	Positioning the hands:	
2	Position the fingers.	
3	Position the transducer.	Is it lying without angulation and parallel to the pads at the side of the table?
4	Position the wrists.	Lay the right wrist along the side pad to facilitate management of the ultrasound probe.
	Manual procedure:	
5	Sliding the probe	Forwards and backwards to identify the hip joint.
6	'Fine tuning'	Small alterations to the transducer position to pinpoint the inferior border of the iliac bone.
7	Freeze the image.	Check whether the correct plane of section has been achieved, showing the inferior tip of the ilium, the labrum and the flat iliac wing. If not, continue:
8	Rotation	Correction of the plane of section.
9	Unfreeze the image.	
10	Repeat from (5) above.	This repetitive motion produces the sequence 'forwards – backwards – fine tuning – stop', followed if necessary by further rotation of the probe.

2. Rotating the probe. The probe is then rotated around the inferior border of the iliac bone, and the image is unfrozen and the technique recommended to obtain the correct plane of section as described in Chapter 7. The examiner can follow the approximate plane of section visually by watching the position of the linear probe head. These situations are shown in Fig. 11.1b to d.

One well-known difficulty occurs when the examiner cannot find the front two-thirds of the acetabular roof. All that can be seen is an iliac contour that runs forwards and appears to represent the oblique edge of a dysplastic socket, and cannot be made to lie parallel to the edge of the image. It is possible in this case that the examiner has made the mistake of taking a section rotated too far forward. This error can be avoided by systematically first finding the posteriorly rotated section showing the concavity of the gluteal fossa (see chapter 7) and then turning the cut further forwards. The concavity will transmute into an oblique line (with the iliac contour running forwards) only after passing through a stage of being parallel to the lateral edge of the image.

If in addition one uses the aid of the echogenicity of the acetabular fossa for fine differentiation, the ideal topographical arrangement of the sections can be achieved with almost millimetre accuracy. As noted in chapter 7, it is unimportant whether the section is taken through the front or the rear part of the acetabular fossa, as long as it is truly coronal.

This repetitive process of homing in on the correct plane of section can be remembered as '*forwards – backwards – fine tuning – stop.*' Each cycle is completed by renewed identification of the inferior point of the ilium, freezing of the picture and checking of the plane of section and the labrum. For further clarity, the main points of the procedure are summarised in Table 11.1.

Key points

- A standard routine is necessary for reliable and reproducible production of standard images.

- The best way to control the child is lying on his side in a specially-designed cradle.

- The probe should be held and moved by a standard technique summarised in Table 11.1.

12 Statistics, clinical findings and therapeutic implications

The results given below are based on a large scientific literature. Note that there are naturally regional variations, especially in the rates of dysplasia, and that more recent investigations are more accurate than earlier ones because of the continuing development of hip sonography.

12.1 Sonographic typing of hips

Dislocation of the hip is the commonest congenital deformity of the locomotor system. In Central Europe it appears in 1-5% of births (Batory 1982, Mau 1983, Bosselmann 1984, Geckeler 1988, Katthagen et al 1986). Estimates of the frequency of hip type I in the neonatal population are shown in Table 12.1. They vary from 56% to 81.1%: other authors give results which lie between these values (Graf 1986, de Jong 1987, Knapp-Birzle 1989). Merk (1992) found 2.53% of all neonatal hip joints to be definitely in need of treatment.

Type Ib occurs 6–7 times more frequently than type Ia: the relative frequencies of these types among all hips studied have been estimated at 69.6% and 9.4% respectively (Graf, 1987), and at 77.9% and 6.4% (Pauer et al., 1988).

12.1.1 Frequency of pathological findings in high-risk groups

A review of the literature giving the frequency of Graf hip types in various clinical groups and various ages is shown in Table 12.2.

Risk factors in general

When children are examined who have predominantly high risk factors and abnormal clinical findings, the rate of dysplasia rises further (Langer 1986, Schober 1990). Prevalences of pathology have been estimated at: 25% pathological sonographic hip types among children with risk factors (Weickert and Merk, 1985),

Table 12.1. Frequency of normal hips (type I) in the general neonatal population. Note also further references in the text

Frequency of type I hips/%	Investigator	Year	Notes
56	Rabenseifner et al.	1987	General neonatal population
56	Oberthaler et al.	1988	
74.4	Dorn et al.	1987	
81.1	Schuler	1988	
59.5	Graf	1990	Infants under 3 months
84.5	Graf	1990	Infants over 3 months

Table 12.2. Review of the literature: Frequencies of hip types (Graf method) in children of various age groups

Author	Year	Number of hip joints	Age	Hip type					
				Ia/Ib	IIa	IIb	IIc/D	IIIa, IIIb	IV
				Frequency in percent					
Bährens	1988	300	<6 wks	93.3	5.3	—	0.66	0.66	—
Bährens	1988	1308	1 d–1 yr	91.8	5.53	1.23	1.07	0.76	0.15
Brackmann et al.	1987	394	<12 wks	65.8	23.4	—	—	10.2	3.6
Eller u. Katthagen	1987	121	>6 wks	—	24.8	49.6	13.2	5.8	—
Gluch u. Skripitz	1988	204	>3 mo	76.0	—	10.3	1.5	0.5	2.9
Godolias	1990	8200	1 d–1 yr	70.05	20.00	1.18	7.65	1.02	0.10
Graf	1986	3104	1 d–1 yr	79.0	8.7	9.9	1.9	0.5	0.1
Graf	1989	3104	75% > 3 mo	77.72	12.28	—	—	—	—
Graf	1990	6754	<3 mo	59.5	35.4	—	4.0	1.0	0.1
Graf	1990	6754	>3 mo	85.4	—	13.2	1.2	0.3	—
Hien et al.	1988	1586	1 d–1 yr	73.6	19.3	4.5	1.7	0.6	0.1
Knapp-Birzle	1989	1900	4,1 mo	73.2	11.8	10.4	1.6	1.5	1.5
Langer	1986	2280	<3 mo	93.2	5.8	—	0.1	0.8	0.1
Oberthaler et al.	1988	846	1–5 d	66.0	31.0	—	2.5	0.5	—
Pauer et al.	1988	1634	1–56 d	29.5	60.3	—	8.3	1.8	0.1
Schuler	1987	1264	7 mo	81.1	8.3	3.2	4.3	2.8	0.2
Schuler	1988		ca. 7 mo	89.4	10.6				
Schwarzkopf	1989	780	ca. 3 mo	44.98	23.13	20.82	5.90	4.12	1.02
Wiese	1986	2608	2.5 mo	90.4	5.7	—	—	2.6	1.3

27% of joints requiring treatment in a group of secondarily referred children (Graf, 1990),

20% of hips requiring treatment in children with a high incidence of historical risk factors and abnormal clinical findings (Weikert and Merk, 1985).

12.2 Historical risk factors and hip sonography

12.2.1 Breech presentation

This is the strongest risk factor for hip abnormalities.

A summary of the literature is given in Table 12.3. See also Breitenfelder (1988), Feltes (1987), Hansson (1988), and Schuler (1988). Between 8.8% and 30% of babies born by breech delivery may have abnormalities of the hips; overall there is a highly sig-

nificant statistical correlation (Table 12.3). This great variation has been explained by the greater number of children with flexed breech presentation in those series showing the lowest numbers of abnormalities. In the extended breech position, the extreme bending of the hips brings pressure to bear upon the dorso-cranial edge of the acetabulum in utero, thus causing deformity of the cartilaginous acetabular rim and limitation of ossification.

Dorn (1990) has commented upon the lesser importance of foot and transverse presentations in predicting pathological hip findings.

12.2.2 Other anamnestic risk factors

Schuler (1988) found that 17% of patients with abnormal hips had a positive *family history*, making this the second most signifi-

Table 12.3. Correlation between breech presentation and abnormality of the hip: overview of the literature. ↑ = significantly raised

Author	Year	No. of infants	% with abnormal hips	Notes
Weikert and Merk	1985		↑	
Rabenseifner et al.	1988	No correlation with breech presentation shown		
Schuler	1988	1264	15	
Schwaberger	1988		30	
Dorn et al.	1988	3047	↑	Extended breech delivery
Ebner	1988		↑	Flexed breech delivery
Dorn	1990	187	8.82	Control group (normal delivery) showed prevalence of 1.81%
Merk	1992	199	26.4	

cant predictor of dysplasia. Other authors have confirmed this result (Rabenseifner et al. 1987, Schwaberger et al. 1988).

Only sporadic reports are available for the other known risk factors (Langer 1986, Menucha 1987, Oberthaler 1987). Neither twins or multiple births, nor premature birth, have been shown to be associated with abnormal hips (Witt et al., 1986; Handel, 1988).

12.3 Clinical findings and hip sonography

12.3.1 Instability of the hip

The literature shows a wide variation in the proportions of clinically normal hips found to be dysplastic at ultrasound, from 1.8% to 50% (Table 12.4). Other authors have recorded the clinical findings in groups of children with sonographically abnormal hips (Table 12.5). 62%–98.7% of such hips have shown clinical signs, and thus 1.3%–38% of sonographically abnormal hips were clinically silent. This broad spectrum has many causes. First, the reliability of the clinical examination is influenced by the age spectrum of the clinical material: hip instability can only be diagnosed with ease within the first few days of life. Secondly, Dorn (1990) has shown a statistical correlation between falling reliability of the examination and increasing number of doctors on the maternity unit. Dunstmann and Gordolias (1988), like other authors, have pointed out that even experienced observers may not be able

Table 12.4. Clinical findings and hip sonography (1): the sensitivity of normal clinical examination

Author	Year	Percentage of clinically normal hips found to be dysplastic	Comments
Clark	1986		
Benz-Bohm	1987	1.8	
Godolias	1990	13.11	4100 children of various age groups studied
Castelein et al.	1988	13.8	
Schwaberger	1988	16	632 neonates studied
Altenhuber et al.	1988	50	
Rabenseifner	1987	50	

Table 12.5. Overview of the literature: Correlation of abnormal clinical findings with abnormal sonography

Author	Year	Percentage of sonographically abnormal hips showing clinical signs	Comments
Eller and Katthagen	1987	76.9	
Merk	1987	61.9	
Schuler	1987	94	
Dorn	1991	98.7	

Table 12.6. Overview of the literature: specificity of positive clinical findings in predicting abnormal ultrasound findings

Author	Year	Percentage of clinically abnormal hips with abnormality at sonography	Comments
Schuler	1987	58	
Ebner	1988		
Eiermacher	1988		
Merk	1985		
Pauer et al.	1988		
Dorn	1991	44.9	Positive Ortolani sign used as criterion
Merk	1992	67.7	120 patients with positive Ortolani sign
Graf et al.	1993	100	41 patients with a positive Barlow test

to recognise clinical instability of the hip. We have been able to see slight clinical instability manifested in the sonogram as clear dislocation.

However, almost all authors agree that real clinical instability is a significant predictor of pathological findings on ultrasound (Table 12.6); other authors have shown that 45%–67.7% of children with clinically abnormal hips or a positive Ortolani sign had abnormal ultrasound findings, and we found that all of 41 patients we studied with a positive Barlow test had abnormal ultrasounds.

12.3.2 Other clinical findings

The prognostic significance of other clinico-pathological findings in the current literature is much more at variance (Dorn 1991, Graf 1991, Schuler 1988, Tönnis 1986, Tschauner 1986, Weber 1988, Weitzel 1987). Schuler (1988) found abnormalities in 30% of patients with *limitation of abduction*. However, most authors consider that isolated limitation of abduction to be non-specific or associated with a normal sonogram (Rabenseifner et al., 1987, Stein and Merk 1987, Merk 1988, Graf 1989).

Asymmetry of the groin folds as an isolated clinical sign can nowadays be disregarded as having any significance for hip dysplasia or hip instability (Schuler 1988, Wetzel 1985, Zick 1987, Zwierchowski 1987). The same is true for *other clinical signs* such as leg shortening, the appearance of asymmetry in the contour of the leg, or external rotation of the limb.

The available studies therefore show that findings at hip sonography correlate only with real clinical instability (the Ortolani 'clunk' and the Barlow subluxation test).

12.4 Hip sonography and the radiograph

As has been noted before, ossifying structures tend to have been visible at sonography for at least 4–6 weeks before they appear on the radiograph. This is because they must be calcified to be visible on the radiograph, and the processes of organisation and ossification in hyaline cartilage produce echoes while they still do not have enough calcification to cause a radiographic shadow. This has to be taken into account when comparing sonograms and radiographs taken at the same time.

The literature contains very few comparisons of radiography with hip sonography (Graf, 1990, Schober, 1990, Weber, 1985). There are probably two reasons for this. One is the difference in the time-scales of use of the two modalities: sonography is mostly used in the first weeks of life, but radiography only has diagnostic value from the fourth month onwards. Secondly, radiography is increasingly being abandoned altogether in favour of sonography except in unclear cases.

Using radiography as the standard procedure, Van Moppers (1986) found that sonography had a sensitivity of 100% and a specificity of 95%. Weber (1987) and Gluch (1988) confirmed this, with 93% and 95.7% agreement between the two modalities. However, Loer et al, (1988) found only 84.8% correlation of the two diagnostic methods. In this study 12.4% of the hips examined had a normal radiograph but a pathological sonographic finding. In 2.7% there was a normal sonographic finding in the presence of a pathological radiograph. Graf (1988, 1989 and 1990) repeatedly demonstrates the higher specificity and sensitivity of sonography.

12.4.1 Are radiographs necessary at all?

This has not been answered satisfactorily (Baehrens, 1988, Sterr, 1989, Zieger, 1986). Eimermacher (1988) and Casser (1987) demand a radiograph at the completion of every treatment, but Graf (1989) only considers this necessary after aggressive therapy continued for several months.

Sonography gives overall much more information than a radiograph. However, radiography may show some bony details better such as necrosis of the femoral head. In view of this, we recommend that a radiograph should be taken:

(a) At the completion of several months of aggressive therapy in order to rule out necrosis of the femoral head,
(b) In cases of insufficient sonographic diagnosis or uncertainty,
(c) If increasing ossification starts to conceal the inferior end of the iliac bone and thus makes sonography useless. See also § 5.2.3.

12.4.2 The radiographic acetabular angle and the bony angle α on the sonogram

Loer in 1988 compared the acetabular angle with the α angle in 185 hip joints. He found a good correlation between the two measured angles. Also, Gluch in 1988 observed an increased number of appearances of pathological acetabular angles in the presence of pathological α angles. He examined 204 hip joints. Our results confirm the reports of both authors. We compared the α angle and the radiographic acetabular angle in 1,824 hip joints and proved a strong indirect relationship between them (r = 0.91).

Table 12.7 shows the results reached by Merk for the sensitivity and specificity of the three most important diagnostic modalities in the infant hip.

Table 12.7. Sensitivity and specificity of diagnostic modalities in the infant hip joint (n = 1824)

Diagnostic modality	Sensitivity in percent	Specificity in percent
Sonography	98.2	99.3
Radiography	92.6	96.5
Clinical diagnosis	39.6	82.2

Table 12.8. Radiography and sonography: Comparison of the methods: the literature and our own results

Author	Year	Correlation in percent
Gluch	1988	95.7
Löer	1988	96.03
Hien	1988	96.03
Schwaberger	1988	84.0
Merk	1992	96.4

12.4.3 Tönnis's classification of subluxation and hip type

There are few references comparing hip sonography with other imaging modalities. In the papers available, plain radiography is used as the 'gold standard'. In Table 12.8 results of representative studies are compared. The agreement between radiography and ultrasonography in establishing Tönnis's hip types varies from 84% to 96.4%.

We used a χ^2 test to compare the distributions of the normal and abnormal findings at radiography and on ultrasound, and found no significant difference (probability of error p = <0.05). This is in good agreement with the other authors quoted.

The appearance of varying findings by comparison of the two methods is not in any way to be blamed upon one or other of the methods. Graf (1987) emphasised the variation in the demonstration of the infant hip in both imaging methods. On the other hand hip sonography shows ossification in the area of the acetabular rim earlier in the timescale than does plain radiography. Due to this alone it is possible that borderline normal hip joints can appear on the radiograph taken at the same time to have hip dysplasia.

Table 12.9 makes clear that because of this, slightly more pathological findings appear on the radiograph than on the ultrasound picture.

Further grounds for the difference may be found in our works and those of Löer (1988) and Schober (1990). Children after ten months of age have a strikingly narrow borderline area for their acetabular angle (method of Tönnis and Brunken), so that dysplastic values of the angle may appear often from this age onwards.

100% correlation of a grade of subluxation has not been found with any particular hip type. The classification systems do not match well, since on the radiological evaluation we only have five grades of subluxation (including the normal situation) to choose from and we have to correlate these with 10 different hip types.

Table 12.9. Comparative evaluations of the sonographic and radiographic findings in the whole clinical material (n = 1824) (Graf 1987)

Findings	Sonographic findings		Radiographic findings	
	Total	Relative frequency	Total	Relative frequency
Pathological	488	26.75	510	27.96
Physiological/normal	1336	73.25	1314	72.04

12.5 Organisation of hip sonography and sonographic follow-up

12.5.1 The maturation curve
(Fig. 12.1)

Longitudinal investigations of the α angle have shown how it varies with age (Tschauner et al., 1992). The shape of this curve allows conclusions to be drawn about the potential for ossification in the acetabular roof. The main thing it shows is that the hip joint shows an enormous potential in the first six weeks of life, which is still present in the second six-week period but reduces considerably after twelve weeks and approaches a level by sixteen weeks with very little movement thereafter. This experience tallies also with the clinical observation that even dislocated joints which receive therapy in the first six weeks, show a very good tendency to heal: indeed the rate of healing is 100% among type IIc hips.

12.5.2 Neonatal screening (Fig. 12.2)

Problems of morbidity due to dysmaturity of the hip can be solved by instituting a general screening programme for all neonates, region by region. Almost without exception, all authors advocate national screening programmes. The only exceptions are those authors who confine their observations to the sonographic diagnosis of subluxed joints (Clark 1987). Taking the growth potential of the infant hip into consideration, the initial examination must take place by the sixth week of life at the latest. Cases requiring treatment may then receive it immediately. A second examination is to be highly recommended during the third to fourth month. At this time, joints found to be immature at the first examination may have their maturity checked for safety's sake, and on the other hand, diagnostic uncertainties at the first examination can be caught. This system forms a reliable safety net for the problem of immaturity of the hip.

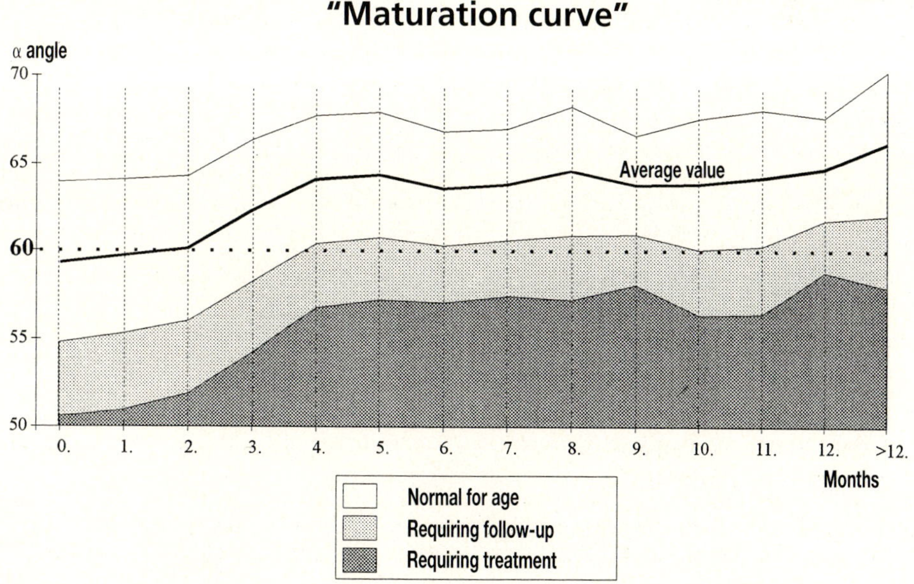

Fig. 12.1. To show the maintenance of the α angle in a longitudinal study of healthy infants. The follow-up zone lies outside one standard deviation of the mean, the treatment zone outside two standard deviations

Incorporation of ultrasound examination into prophylactic care

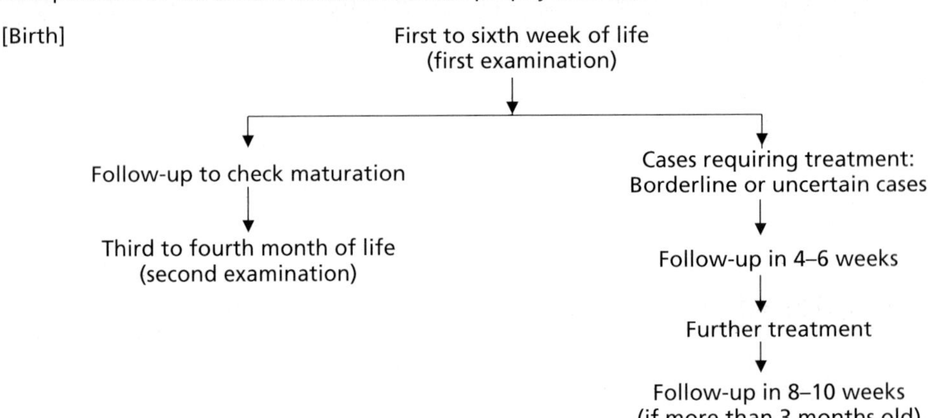

Fig. 12.2. Scheme of examinations for screening and treating cases

12.5.3 Follow-up intervals

Because of the growth potential of the hip joint, joints that are younger than three months old and requiring treatment should be followed up in four to six weeks. In babies older than three months, the potential for growth slows down considerably so that a follow-up interval of eight to 10 weeks is in order. (The earlier rule to keep on following up hips by sonograpy until the ossification centre of the femoral capital epiphysis appears, is thought to be superfluous in the current state of the art.)

12.5.4 Premature infants

Newborn infants do indeed show an increased rate of immaturity of their hips, but no increased rate of pathology when the degree of prematurity of birth is taken into account. Our own investigations have shown that hips that require treatment at birth show a disproportionate degree of healing by the sixth week. The classification of prematurely born hip joints is discussed in chapter 8.

Key points

- Several risk factors for dysplasia of the hip have been identified. These include:
  Breech presentation (especially extended breech)
  Family history
  Clinical instability of the hip

- Sonograms have been shown to give much more information in the first three months of life than radiographs do.

- Radiographs may only be needed on rare occasions.

- Because of the different information given by ultrasound and radiography, there is rather poor correlation between ultrasound findings and Tönnis's classification of subluxation.

- Neonatal screening programmes are the best way to reduce morbidity from congenital dislocation of the hip.

13 Sonographic control of therapy

13.1 Principles of treatment

Experience in the treatment of hip dysplasias and luxations from the literature, together with our experience of hip sonography, and histological and morphological studies, allow important principles to be identified:

1. Therapy should be initiated in the important period up to the sixth week of life, to exploit the optimal growth potential at that time. The investigations of Barlow (1962) and von Rosen (1969) showed that if disturbances of the hip maturation can be recognised immediately after birth and if adequate treatment is started immediately, an almost complete anatomical healing can be accomplished, and this remains the main aim of treatment. According to Becker (1979) and Schultheiss (1965), complete healing can only be attained in about two thirds of cases if treatment is delayed until after the first three months of life.

Many reports in the literature confirm that the age at diagnosis can be brought forward considerably by sonographic examination. There is also unanimous agreement that early diagnosis can shorten and simplify treatment. The number of operations on the infant hip joint sinks (Graf, 1990).

2. Compressive, distractive and shearing forces on the acetabular roof bring growth and ossification of the acetabular roof to a standstill, and in addition lead to histological deformation (degeneration) of the hyaline cartilaginous part of the acetabular roof, as in type IIIb hips.

Application of these principles in a firmly defined therapeutic protocol has meant that:

1. Even dislocated joints can be restored and healed with conservative therapy alone by an average age of 7.5 months,

2. Necrosis of the femoral head can be completely avoided.

These results are encouraging but show that a review of treatment techniques is necessary if further improvement is to be obtained.

Every successful treatment depends upon knowledge of the prevailing patho-anatomical situation of the joint, and the recognition that every treatment method and every orthosis has a quite specific biomechanical function; these are given in more detail below. So for example, a dislocated hip joint should not be treated with an abduction harness which is designed biomechanically as an orthosis for late maturation. It would be equally senseless to treat a Type IIb joint (a simple dysplasia) with overhead extension. Arbitrary mixing of the treatment methods and uncritical use can only lead to failure. Treatment methods that can in certain circumstances function in all three phases (e.g. the Pavlik harness) require to be strictly supervised as they have to be repeatedly readjusted according to the various phases of treatment.

13.2 Phases of treatment

Each joint lies in a quite definite (pathological) biomechanical situation according to its sonographic type. In order to be able to react with a corresponding biomechanical mode of therapy, an exact sonographic examination must first of all be carried out to assess the condition of the hip.

13.2.1 Reduction phase

(Fig. 13.1a to c)

In dislocated joints (types D, IIIa, IIIb, IV) the first necessary step in treatment is to reduce the femoral head as far as the true acetabulum. Not all equipment available on the market is equally suitable for reduction of the hip. Some of the means of treatment appear as examples in table 13.1.

We ourselves prefer relocation by overhead extension ('gallows') traction. From the biomechanical standpoint it is irrelevant for the hip whether overhead traction is used immediately or whether it follows longitudinal traction. If gallows traction is used, in no case should it reach more than 45° to 50° of abduction. When the diagnosis has been made very early (before the sixth week) extension traction is not usually required, as the femoral head is spontaneously relocatable. Dynamic sonography can be used to tell whether the joint is spontaneously relocatable and/or whether overhead extension traction is necessary.

In principle it is enough to place the dislocated femoral head against the mouth of

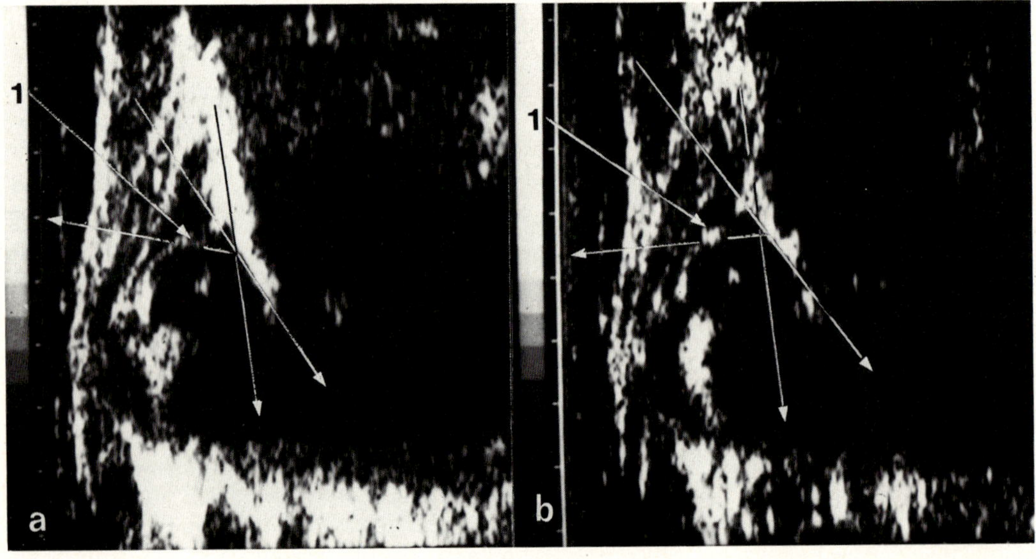

Fig. 13.1a. Four-week-old baby with poor bony formation. The bony rim is flattened, the cartilaginous rim is widened, the labrum is compressed upwards, the hyaline structure is preserved. Acetabular labrum (1). α=25°, β=115°, type IIIa

Fig. 13.1b. The same hip after a week of gallows traction. The α angle has remained the same but the cartilaginous rim is improving and is not compressed as far upwards as in Figure 14.1a. The β angle is now 90°

Fig. 13.1c. Reduction phase. The aim of this phase of treatment is to reduce the femoral head against the true acetabulum, or if possible to place the head right into the hollow of the socket

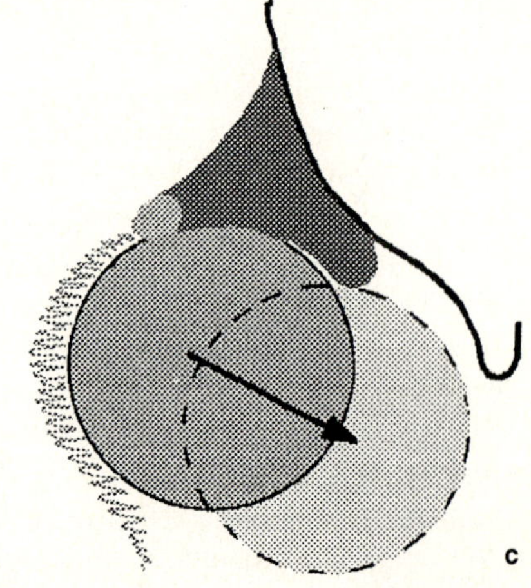

Table 13.1. Treatment concepts

Phase	Hip type	Treatment	Alternative	Remarks
1) Reduction (dislocated joints)	III–IV Type D	Overhead traction or manual reduction (differentiate sonographically)	Reduction orthosis (Pavlik, Hanausek, Düsseldorf, Fettweis splint etc.)	Parental compliance? Ability to follow up?
2) Retention (previously dislocated joints now relocated but unstable)	All relocated joints Unstable type IIc (except for unstable IIc joints in the newborn)	Squatting plaster (ca. 4 weeks)	Retention orthosis (Pavlik, plaster splint, Fettweis orthosis. Düsseldorf splint., etc.	
3) Final maturation (stable, 'dysplastic' joints)	All retained joints	Graf-Mittelmeier abduction harness	Maturation orthosis: splints, abduction harness, Pavlik Bernau, etc.	
	Unstable IIc in the newborn	Graf-Mittelmeier		4 weeks' trial. If stable, continue. If unstable, retention in squatting plaster
	IIa, IIb	Graf-Mittelmeier	Fettweis, Hilgenreiner, Optimal frame, activity abduction harness, etc.	

the true acetabulum. It is often not possible to locate the femoral head deep in the true acetabulum because of the compressed acetabular roof cartilage; this often has to be a dynamic process lasting for several weeks. The reduction phase ends with successful relocation of the femoral head.

13.2.2 Retention phase (Fig. 13.2)

(a) Biomechanical considerations. At this stage the femoral head has been repositioned at the mouth of or within the true acetabulum. However the cartilaginous acetabular roof is still deformed and incongruent, and possesses a secondary depression. The joint capsule is stretched and loose, and the femoral head tends to dislocate again into the secondary depression; it cannot be fixed into the true acetabulum because of the incongruent cartilaginous acetabular roof and the loose capsule, and is therefore still unstable.

(b) Biomechanical principles of treatment. The femoral head must be inserted deep into the socket in order to relieve the pres-

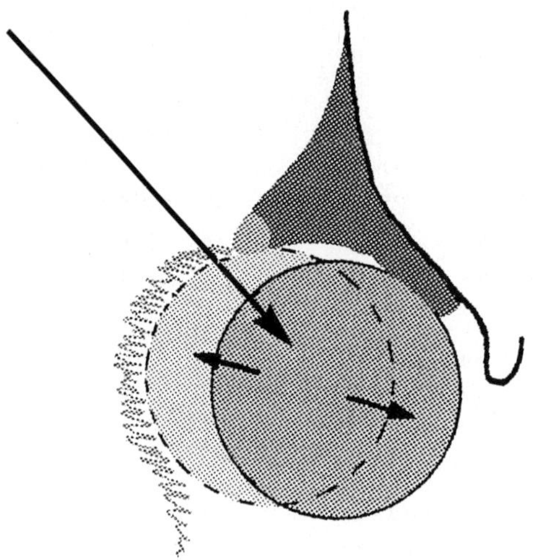

Fig. 13.2. Retention phase. The femoral head is unstable: it can be reduced but tends to reluxate into the pseudo-acetabulum. The cartilaginous roof is still deformed, and the joint capsule is stretched. The required re-insertion of the head deep into the acetabulum is indicated by the large arrow

sure on the cartilaginous acetabular roof. (Remember that pressure on the acetabular roof prevents it from growing.) This deep insertion of the femoral head can be attained by a squatting position or by the so-called foetal position. The legs must be flexed by at least 90°, preferably 100°.

Abduction of over 45° to 50° must be avoided as the axial pressure into the socket rises and the blood vessels can be strained with abduction greater than this.

The joint must be left to rest for a relatively long time in this position so that:

(a) the deformed cartilaginous roof can unfold itself again and can come to lie congruently over the femoral head, and
(b) the loose joint capsule gets a chance to shrink.

The duration appears to depend upon the age of the child and to run from 2–6 weeks with an average of 4 weeks.

In this phase of retention any possibility that the femoral head could slide back and forth in the widened and deformed acetabu-

lum must be completely avoided. Any so-called retention orthosis which is likely to work in this phase must be able to provide deep insertion of the femoral head with a maximum of 45° to 50° abduction and firm fixation in this position. For reasons which we will discuss later, we have gone back to fixation in a sitting plaster spica in preference to other methods. After the time period mentioned, the hip joint enters the late maturation phase.

13.2.3 Late maturation phase
(Fig. 13.3)

Biomechanical situation: The hip joint has been reduced deep in the socket and the cartilaginous acetabular roof has been unfolded and laid congruently over the femoral head. The joint capsule is taut. The hip joint is stable. The cartilaginous acetabular roof however is not yet adequately ossified. The hip joint can be moved once again but pressure on the acetabular roof must be

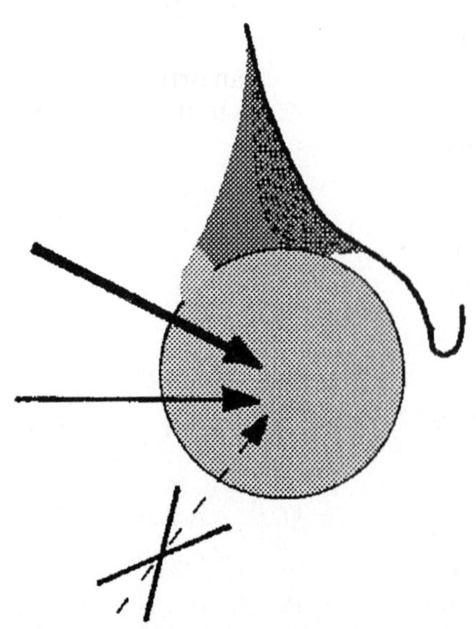

Fig. 13.3. Late maturation phase. Pressure on the area of the acetabular roof must be avoided at all costs. If possible, the head should continue to be inserted deep into the socket but some movement of the joint is allowable

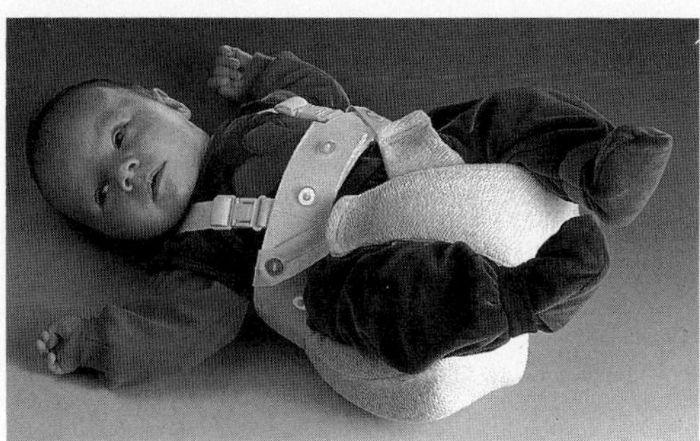

Fig. 13.4. The Mittelmeier-Graf harness as a means of obtaining final maturation. Modified squatting position. Restraining wedges prevent over-abduction. Correct adjustment of the straps according to the patient's size allows for some movement

absolutely avoided because of its influence upon growth and ossification. (Remember the dangers of badly-fitting harnesses in this context. For example, if the abduction bar between the thighs is too short it can allow the femoral heads to remain dislocated within the plaster. This effect may be exacerbated by inadequate flexion.) The sonographic types that require induction of late maturation are Type IIc stable, IIa($-$), and IIb.

To attain this goal an orthosis for maturation needs to conform to these principles (a) movement, (b) at least 90% flexion (a slightly reduced sitting or squatting position), (c) avoidance of abduction over 50°. Typical orthoses for maturation that more or less fulfil these pre-requisites include abduction harnesses (Fig. 13.4).

13.3 Problems in treatment

(a) Treatment planning. It is not good enough to arrive at a correct diagnosis for an infant as late as the sixth week of life. If treatment starts this late then a rapid deterioration of the prognosis can be expected. Similarly, a poor outcome may arise iatrogenically if the treatment has not been clearly and sequentially designed by the medical staff from the start. Thus, an early diagnosis

may be spoilt by misjudgement of the sonographic and pathoanatomical findings in the hip joint which can lead to the wrong method of treatment being chosen. Failure of this may only become apparent in 4–6 weeks, and modification of treatment will then be too late to catch the optimal time period. Such a 'trial and error' method is to be deprecated.

(b) Compliance. Even when a correct and early diagnosis and treatment plan have been formulated, the parents may for various reasons not be able to manage the chosen treatment. Alteration, removal or maladjustment of the device, particularly in the retention phase, can be catastrophic for the joint. In order to render this problem of compliance and treatment independent of parental influence, we have fallen back upon fixation in plaster. A plaster cast will not damage the hip unless it is applied in a badly chosen position such as the Lorenz position. The padding under the coils of plaster enable micro-movements to go on so that cartilage nuitrition can continue.

13.3.1 Exceptions in the case of neonates

Neonates in the first ten days of life have an enormous potential for maturation of the hip. Thus, a well- and tightly-fitting abduction harness (a Mittelmeier-Graf harness size 1 with parallel straps) is used in type IIc unstable or type D hips in this group in preference to fixation in plaster. The joint is followed up in four weeks. If the hip has stabilised, treatment principles dictate that it has entered the late maturation phase, and treatment with the abduction harness can be continued. However, if the joint turns out to have been under-treated this way, that is, that no improvement on the initial condition has been obtained and the hip has remained unstable, then rigid fixation in a squatting plaster spica is instituted at once. The hip joint in such cases would still be under the critical age of six weeks.

13.3.2 Age limit

Sonography has to be abandoned at the age when increasing ossification in the femoral head begins to obscure the lower edge of the iliac bone (see § 5.2.3), thus making definition of the standard plane impossible. Our experience has been that hip sonography can be used excellently well from birth to the twelfth month of life. From then on it can indeed be used, but is increasingly overtaken by plain radiography. Even in older children, sonography can be used to judge the growth zone in the acetabular rim in selected cases. This acetabular rim is visible even in older children as it is not covered by any structures which totally reflect the ultrasound beam. The depth of the acetabulum cannot be demonstrated because the bony parts of the femoral head are so well developed. If the problem at issue is simply the degree to which the bony acetabular roof still consists of its cartilaginous model, sonography can succeed in preference to the much more invasive procedure of arthrography.

Key points

- Successful treatment depends upon starting earlier than the sixth week, and avoiding abnormal forces upon the femoral head and acetabular roof.

- Each phase of treatment requires individual assessment and varying therapeutic approaches.

- In the reduction phase, the femoral head is brought down to lie against the orifice of the acetabulum.

- In the retention phase, the femoral head is placed fully home in the acetabulum in order to stabilise it and re-form the cartilaginous acetabular roof.

- In the late maturation phase, the femoral head is held in place while secondary ossification is stimulated in the acetabular roof to allow it to remain fixed in position.

(Not all the examples shown come from joints examined in a routine sonographic screening programme!)

14.1 Hip joint type IIIa; progress under treatment

This twelve day old female baby (I. K.) received routine sonographic screening as a neonate. There was a family history of dysplasia in the mother and clinically an isolated left-sided restriction of abduction could not be excluded with confidence. A dislo-

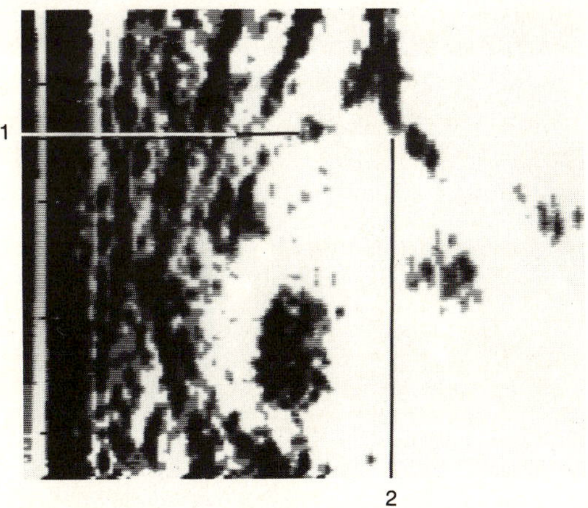

Fig. 14.2. Digitised image of Figure 14.1.

1 Labrum
2 Transition point

The salient points can be brought out even more clearly by digitisation

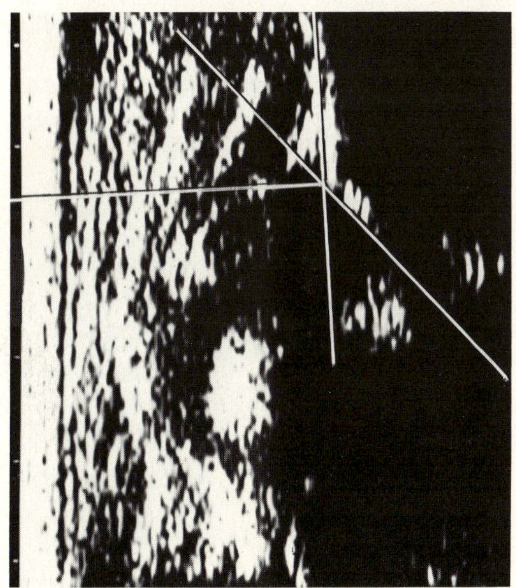

Fig. 14.1. I. K. 12 days old, left hip joint. Poor bony formation. The bony rim is flat. The cartilaginous acetabular roof is widened and pushed cranially but has a normal echo-poor structure. Hip type IIIa. $\alpha = 40°$, $\beta = 90°$

cated hip of hip type IIIa was discovered sonographically (Figs. 14.1, 14.2). The radiograph showed a distinct lateralisation of the upper end of the femur on the left side (Fig. 14.3). Treatment was initiated with fixation of the hip joint in a Fettweis plaster and four weeks later the hip was shown to have stabilised both clinically and sonographically. It was then treated with three months' abduction and in the fourth month of life follow up sonography was carried out (Figs. 14.4, 14.5). The hip is completely correctly roofed over and the bony and cartilaginous relations of the acetabular roof are normal for the child's age, hip type Ia. The treatment with abduction was discontinued. A final checkup at twelve months of age disclosed a clinically completely unremarkable hip entirely compatible with age (Fig. 14.6).

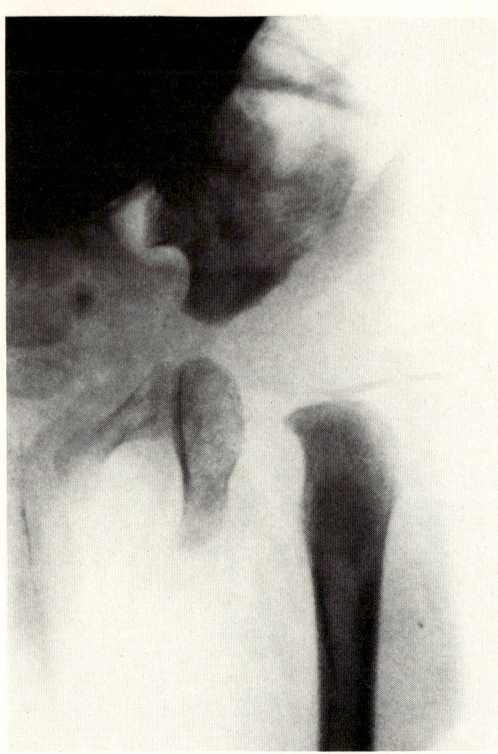

Fig. 14.3. Radiograph to Figures 14.1 and 14.2. Clear lateralisation of the proximal end of the femur and a shallow acetabulum

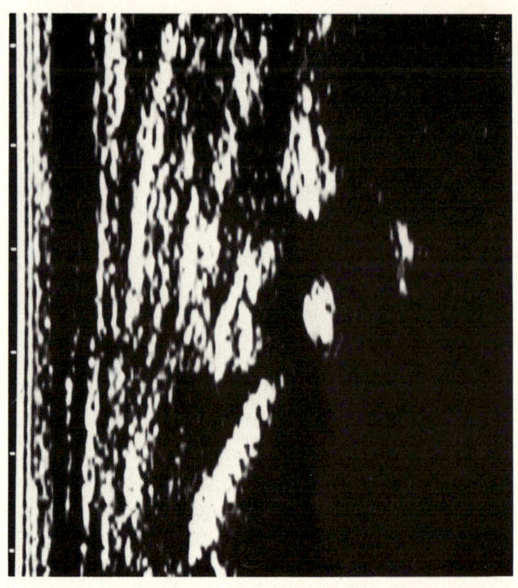

Fig. 14.4. I. K. 4 months old. Left hip joint projected to the right-hand side. Bony formation is very good. The bony rim is angular. Cartilaginous acetabular roof is narrow and overlapping and the femoral head has started to ossify. Hip type I

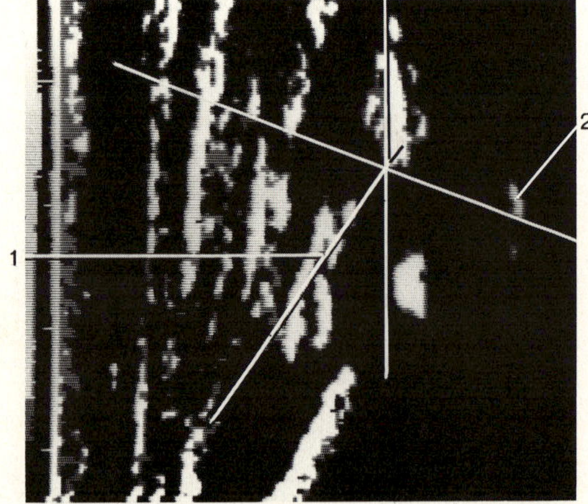

Fig. 14.5. Digitised image of Figure 14.4 with the measurement lines drawn. $\alpha = 68°$, $\beta = 39°$. Hip type Ia.

1 Acetabular labrum
2 Inferior border of the iliac bone

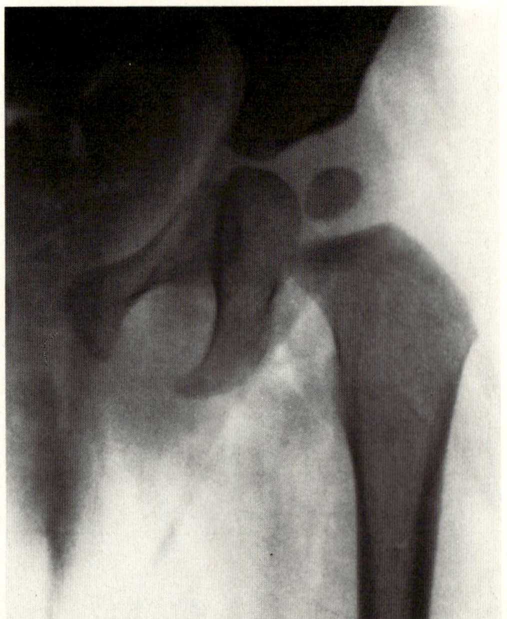

Fig. 14.6. Radiograph of patient I.K. at the age of 12 months. Completely unremarkable radiological findings in the hip joint

14.2 Follow-up of progress patient W. D. Initial findings type IIIa

An eight week old baby is presented who is said to have had normal clinical findings when his hips were routinely examined at birth. The right hip joint was sonographically type I, but the left hip was sonographically type IIIa (Fig. 14.7). Under pressure this hip joint dislocated further (Fig. 14.8); under tension it was possible to draw the femoral head caudally but a genuine reduction of the femoral head was not possible (Fig. 14.9). The corresponding radiograph is shown in Fig. 14.10. In view of the relatively good result of attempted reduction on ultrasound, a squatting plaster was applied.

Eight weeks' fixation in this plaster produced good reduction (Fig. 14.11). The femoral head is centred in a sonographically type IIb joint with a clearly widened cartila-

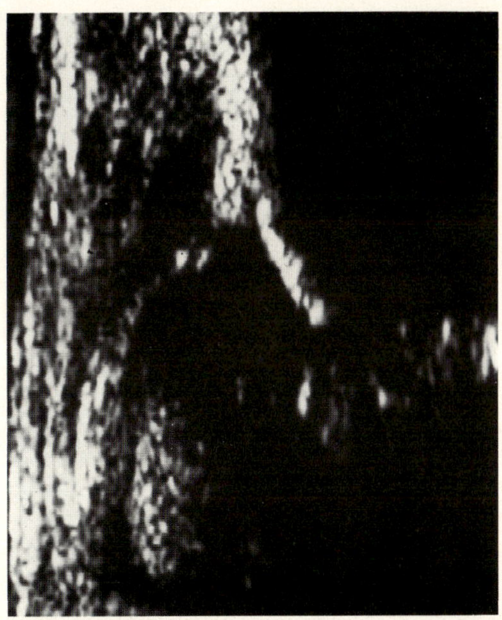

Fig. 14.7. Eight week old left hip. The bony formation is poor, the bony rim is flat. The cartilaginous acetabular roof is compressed cranially and is echo-poor. type IIIa

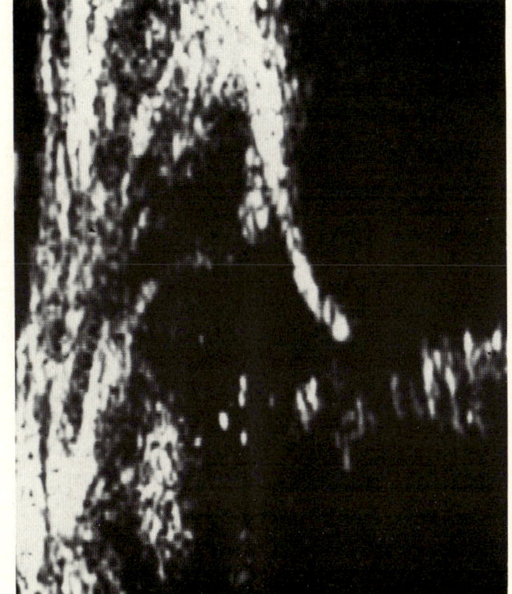

Fig. 14.8. The same hip joint as in 14.7 under compression. The femoral head is clearly dislocated further upwards

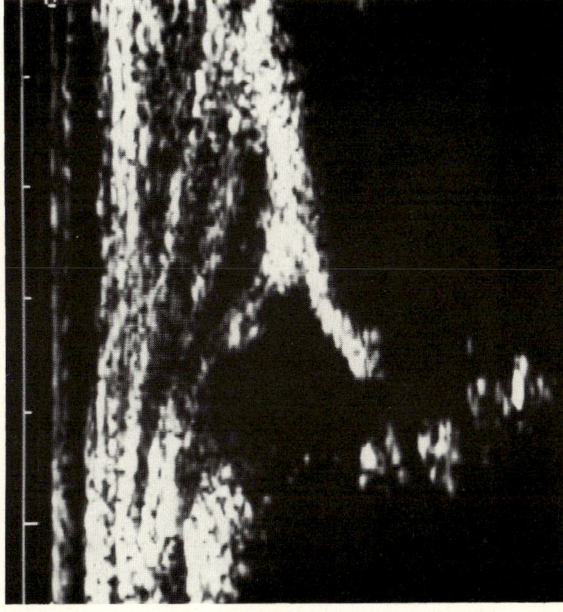

Fig. 14.9. The same hip joint as in Figure 14.7 under tension (attempted reduction). The femoral head slides deeper into the socket but ideal reduction is not possible

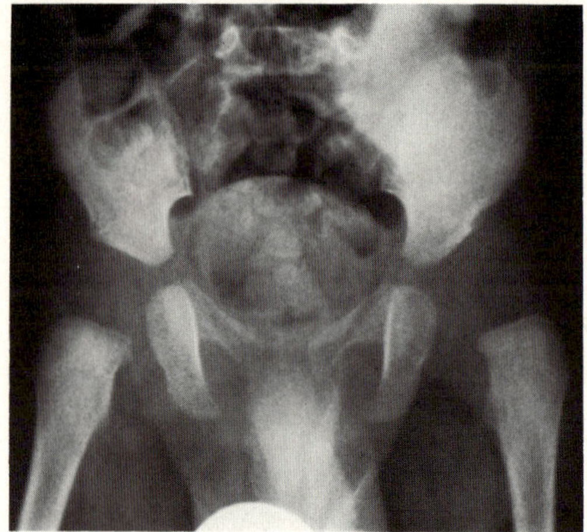

Fig. 14.10. Radiograph to Figure 14.7

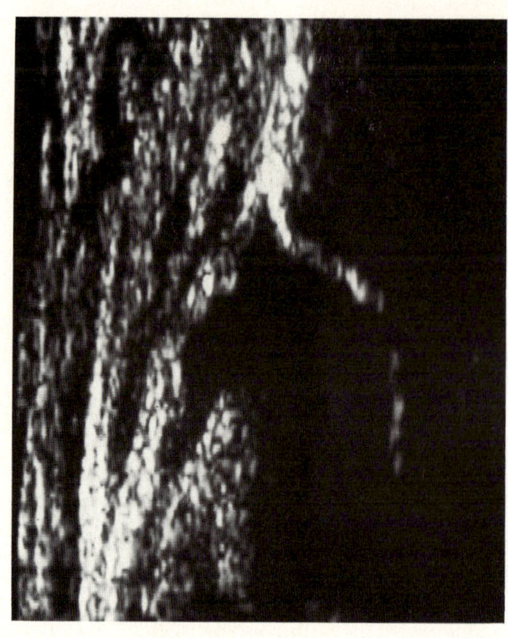

Fig. 14.11. Good relocation after a squatting plaster. type IIb with the cartilaginous roof still clearly widened

ginous acetabular roof. Further treatment followed with a retention splint for three months. After removal of the splint a type I joint was found, still with a widened cartilaginous acetabular roof (Fig. 14.12). Final fol-

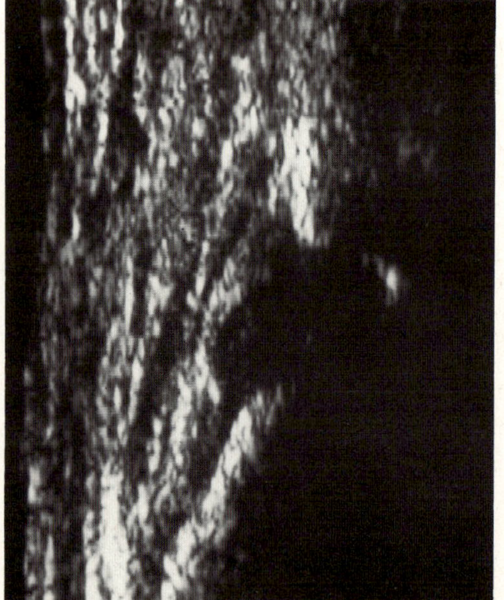

Fig. 14.12. Result after three months' treatment with a retention splint. The bony rim is already well contoured but the cartilaginous acetabular roof is still somewhat wide. Borderline normal finding

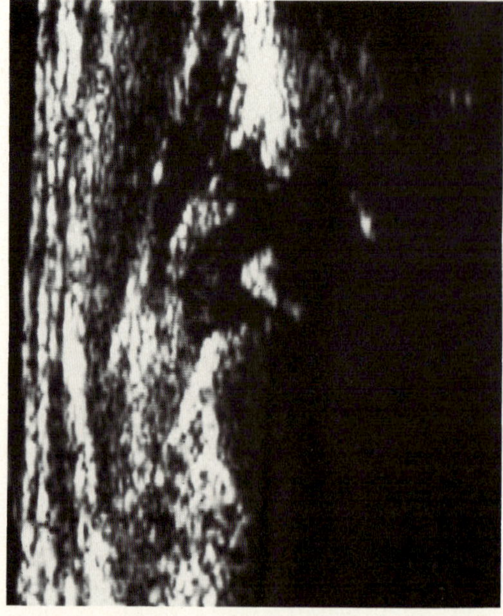

Fig. 14.13. Late follow up after nine months' treatment. The type I joint is seen with ossification in the femoral head and a cartilaginous acetabular roof which is still somewhat widened

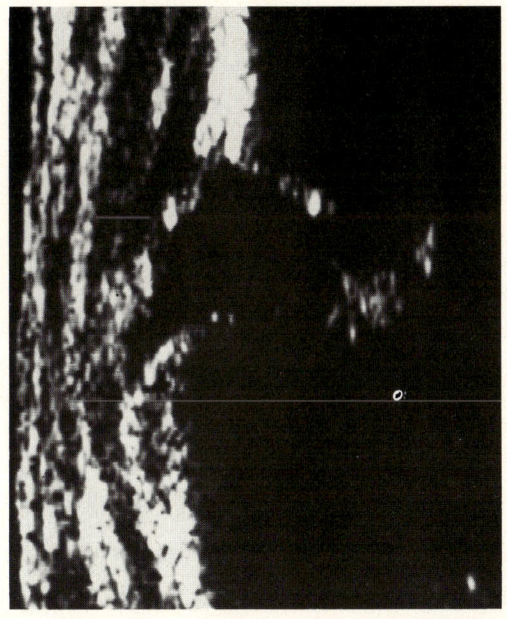

Fig. 14.14. This sonogram (Type I) is an image of the healthy right hip corresponding to the right side of the radiograph in Figure 14.10

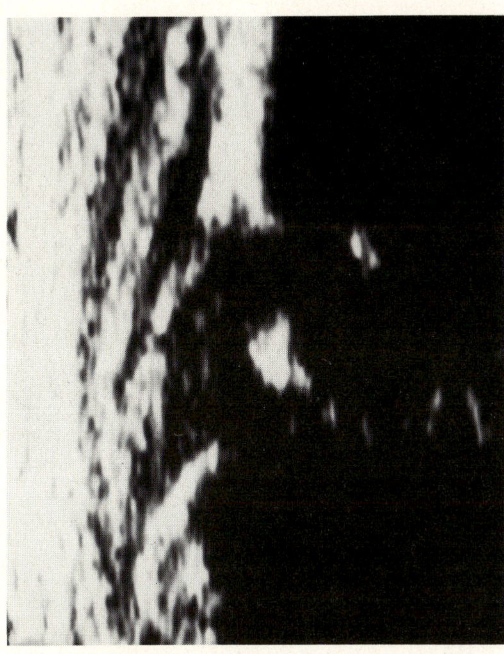

Fig. 14.15. A healthy right hip joint for comparison with Figure 14.13. Type I

low up after nine months shows a completely matured hip joint, type I, with early ossification in the femoral capital epiphysis (Fig. 14.13). For comparison, Fig. 14.14 shows the sonogram of the right hip joint in the same child at the initial examination, corresponding to the radiograph in Fig. 14.10. Fig. 14.13 shows the right hip joint at nine months for comparison with the final mature result on the left side (Fig. 14.15).

14.3 Follow-up for progress with conservative therapy (hip type D)

(Figs. 14.16–14.20)

Baby girl H.A. did not present for her first routine ultrasound examination until the age of three months. The history was unremarkable: the hips had been normal on clinical examination at birth.

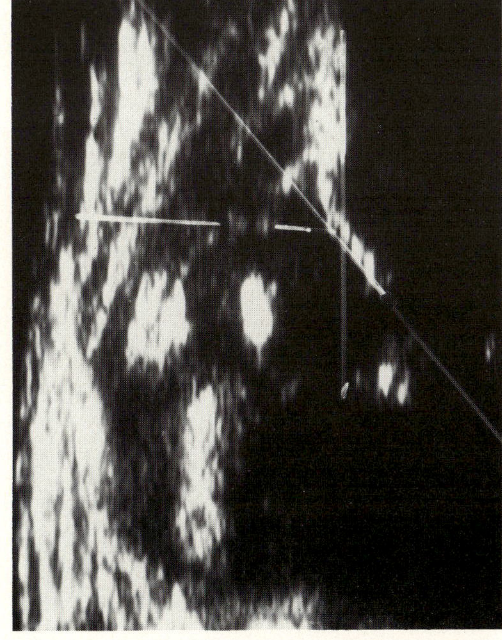

Fig. 14.16. Patient H. A. 3 months old right hip joint. A dislocated joint with hip type D. The measurement lines have been constructed

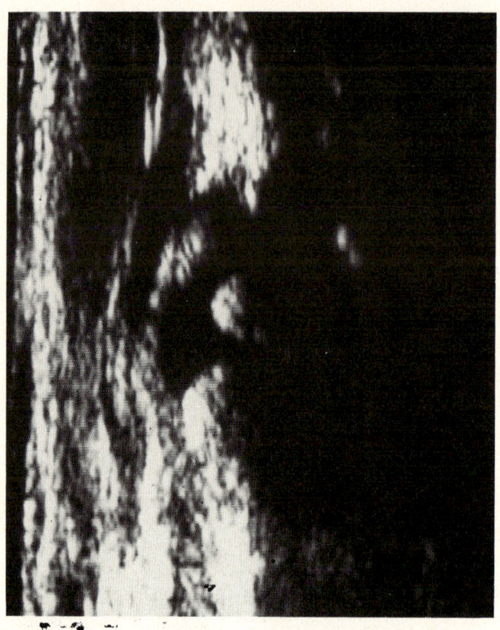

Fig. 14.17. Patient H.A., after 2 months' treatment with a splint in a flexed and abducted position. The hip joint is well centred. Type IIb corresponding to the radiograph in Figure 14.18

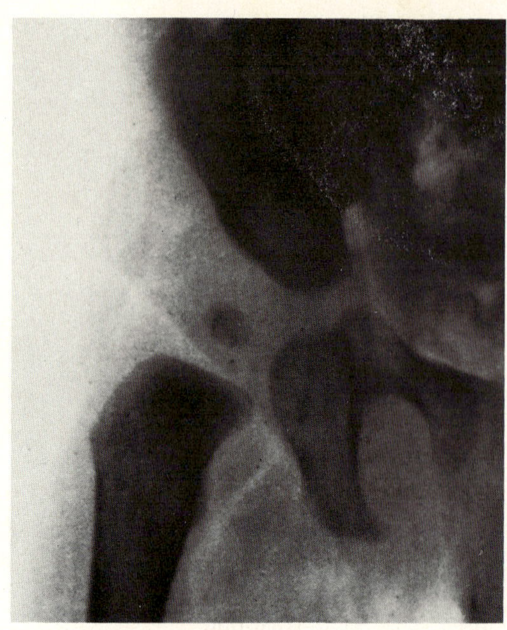

Fig. 14.18. Radiograph corresponding to Figure 14.17

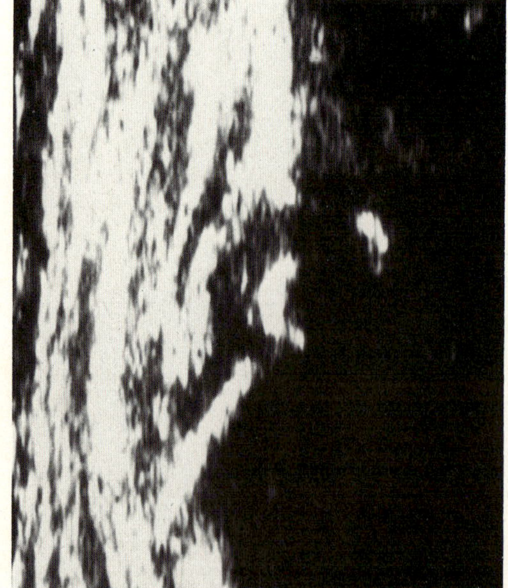

Fig. 14.19. Patient H. A. Well developed result after 7 months' treatment with abduction. A mature hip joint of hip type I corresponding with the radiograph in Figure 14.20

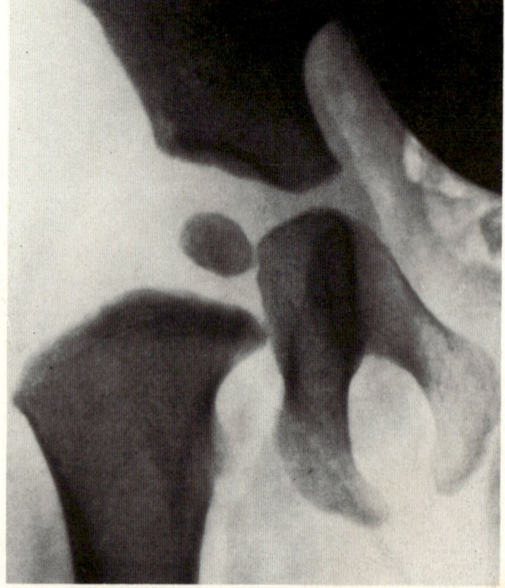

Fig. 14.20. Radiograph to Figure 14.19

However at the first ultrasound examination a hip type D was demonstrated on the right side (Fig. 14.16). Abduction therapy was immediately instituted in a flexed and mildly abducted position for two months and this led to the joint becoming centred (Figs. 14.17 and 14.18).

The mature result after seven months' treatment is shown in Figs. 14.19 and 14.20.

14.4 Follow-up for progress. Hip type IIIb with treatment in a Fettweis plaster

Patient M. E. was referred to us at the age of four months with an isolated limitation of abduction. At ultrasound examination a type IIIb hip was found (Fig. 14.21). The child was treated with a Fettweis plaster over four weeks in order to relieve the load on the acetabular roof by positioning the femoral head deep in the acetabulum. After the plaster was removed he was further treated with a Hilgenrein splint. At the age of 11 months (Fig. 14.22) the bony rim was

sonographically well contoured but the ossified area was still inadequate. The cartilaginous rim was wide but overlapping (type IIb).

At follow up at the age of 2 years there was unfortunately still a residual dysplasia (Fig. 14.23). This confirms our experience of type IIIb hips in similar circumstances: they seem to tend towards a residual dysplasia because of the disturbance in the area of the growth zone in spite of correct and intensive therapy.

14.5 Follow-up for progress of type IIIb hip under therapy

This baby girl was not referred to our department until the age of five months, after failed treatment with an abduction harness. The clinical findings had been unremarkable in the right hip but there was an isolated limitation of abduction on the left. Sonographically a type III hip was shown which already had definite hyperechogenicity of the cartilaginous acetabular roof

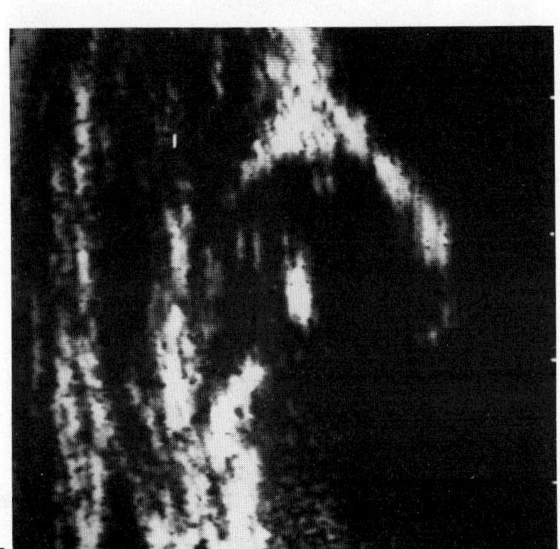
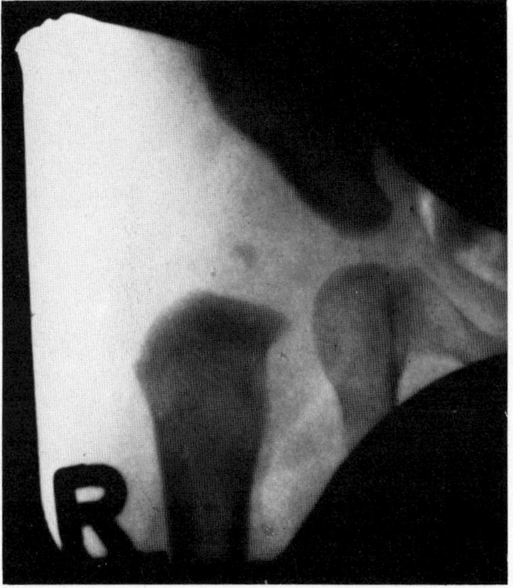

Fig. 14.21a, b. Sonogram of the right hip with its radiograph. The bony formation is poor, the cartilaginous acetabular roof is widened, compressed and echogenic. Type IIIb (four months old)

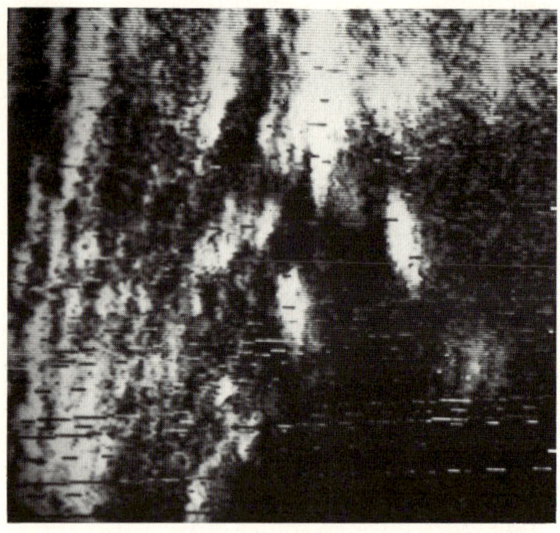

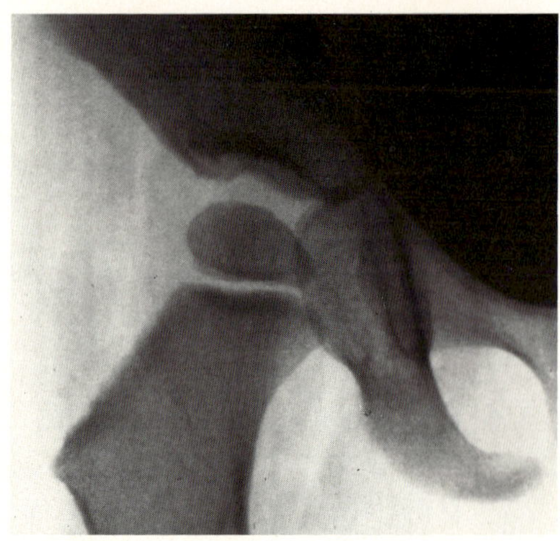

Fig. 14.22. The bony formation is deficient in the presence of good bony contouring of the rim, the cartilaginous rim is somewhat wide but still overlaps and the sonographic structure is normal. Type IIb (11 months old). $\alpha = 55°$, $\beta = 65°$

Fig. 14.23. The same patient as in Figures 14.21 and 14.22. A clear defect in the acetabular rim is demonstrable (2 years of age)

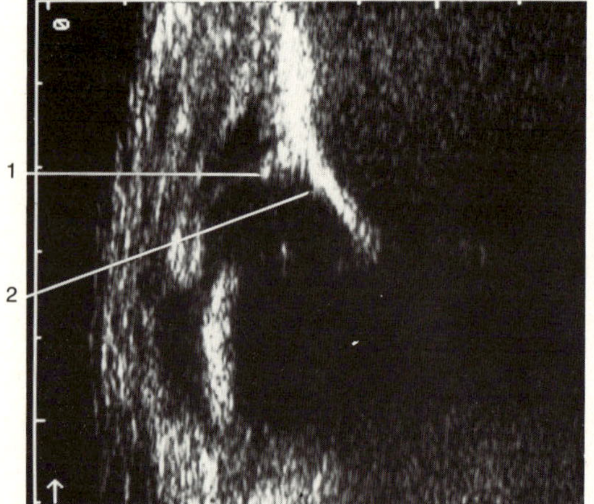

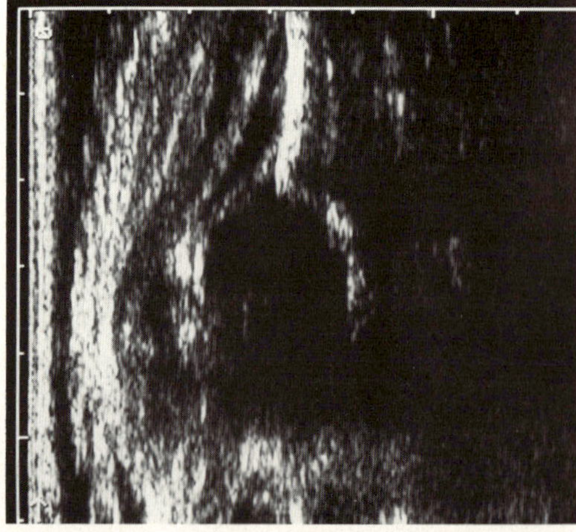

Fig. 14.24. Patient H. N. 5 months old. Left hip joint corresponding to Figure 14.27. The bony formation is poor. The bony rim is flat. The cartilaginous acetabular roof is compressed upwards and increasingly echogenic.

1 Acetabular labrum
2 Bony acetabular rim

Fig. 14.25. H. N. 5 months old. Right hip joint corresponding to Figure 14.26. The bony formation is adequate or good. The bony rim is angular. The cartilaginous acetabular roof is widely overlapping.

$\alpha = 60°$, $\beta = 75°$. Hip type Ib (borderline normal finding)

(Fig. 14.24). The right hip joint was sonographically unremarkable except for a mild delay in ossification (Fig. 14.25). Radiological findings (Figs. 14.26 and 14.27) corresponded to the sonographic findings. On the subluxed left side, a clear lateralisation could be diagnosed with superior displacement of the proximal end of the femur and flattening of the acetabular roof. After three weeks of treatment by extension traction a

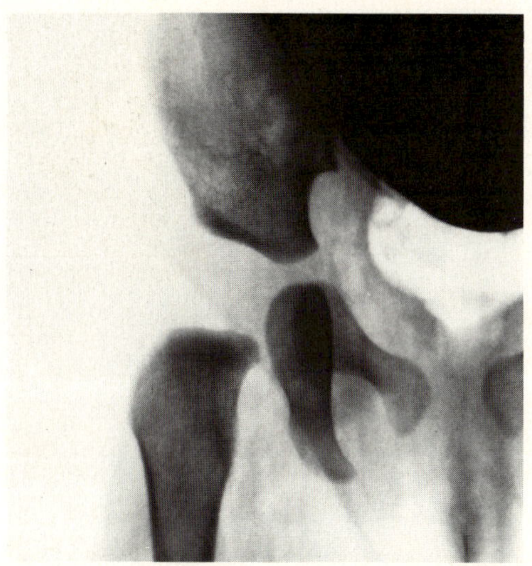

Fig. 14.26. Radiograph to Figure 14.25

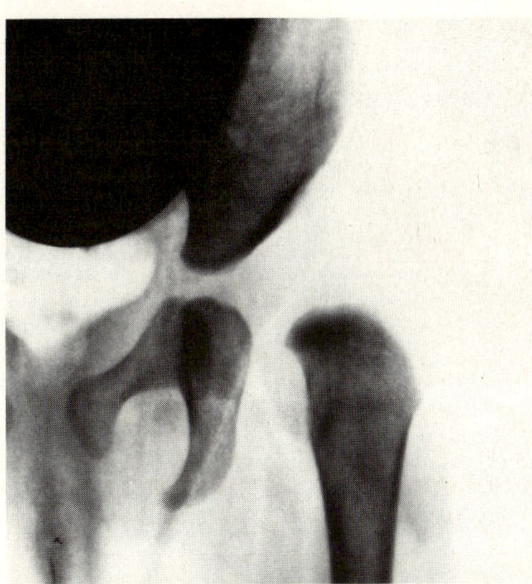

Fig. 14.27. Radiograph to Figure 14.24

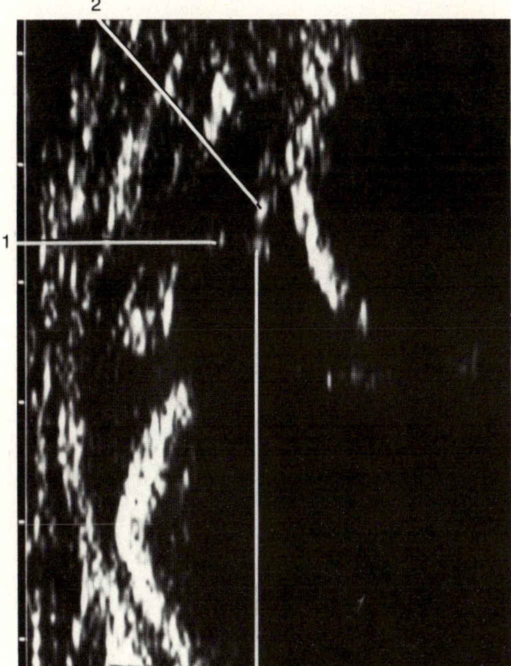

Fig. 14.28. H. N. after longitudinal extension. The bony formation is poor. The bony rim is flattened. The cartilaginous acetabular roof is wide and compressed upwards. Cartilaginous structure is still echo-poor in comparison with Figure 14.24. Hip type IIIa.

1 Acetabular labrum
2 Proximal perichondrium
3 Line of division between the cartilaginous acetabular roof and the femoral head

clear improvement of the structural disturbance in the cartilaginous acetabular roof could be demonstrated on follow-up ultrasound (Fig. 14.28). The cartilaginous acetabular roof seemed to unfold when stretched but was still not clearly compressed proximally (hip type IIIa). Under anaesthesia complete reduction was achieved; the femoral head could be returned to the socket without any problems. After four weeks' fixation in a Fettweis plaster the hip was clinically stable and was further treated with an abduction splint. The result at follow up ultrasound 2 months later can been in Fig. 14.29. The bony formation is however still deficient and the femoral head does not appear to be quite ideally centred. Sonographic overview of the hip joint showed a clear instability. It was therefore necessary to reapply the plaster for a further six weeks and this led to a stabilisation of the hip. However at sonographic control a clear defect in the rim in the middle part of the acetabulum was visible. At a final follow up at thirteen months (Figs. 14.30 and 14.31) a definite delay in ossification could be seen sonographically which corresponds to the severe defect in the bony rim in Fig. 14.31.

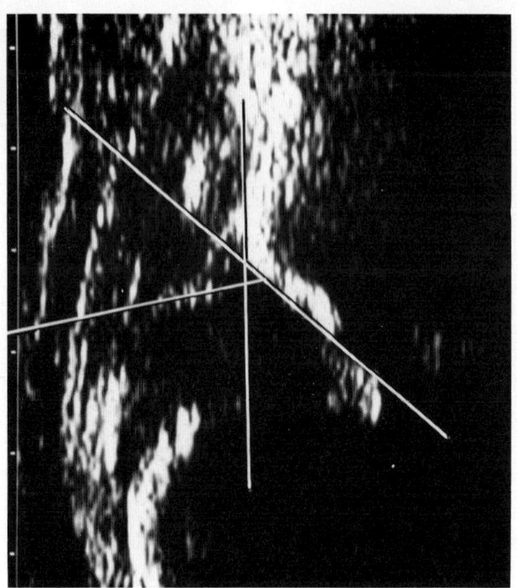

Fig. 14.29. The same hip joint as in Figure 14.28 after premature removal of the plaster at the age of eight months. The bony formation is seriously deficient, the bony rim is rounded. The cartilaginous acetabular roof seems to be widened and compressed. The measurement lines are not correctly applied as this cut was taken somewhat too far dorsally.
$\alpha = 48°$, $\beta = 82°$, hip type D

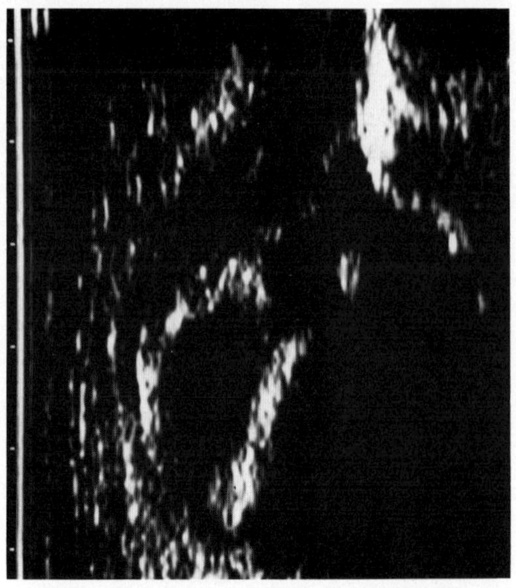

Fig. 14.30. H.N. left hip joint corresponding with the radiograph in Figure 14.31. Bony formation is deficient. The bony rim is rounded. The cartilaginous acetabular roof is badly widened but overlapping. Hip type IIb

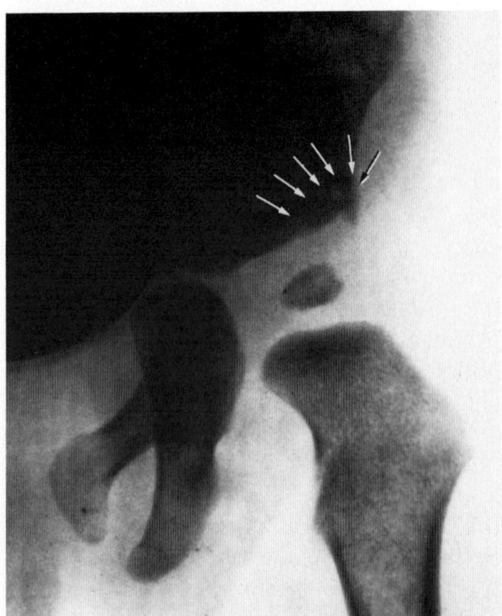

Fig. 14.31. Radiograph to Figure 14.30. The bony roofing of the acetabulum is satisfactory but there is a noticeable defect in the rim which is marked with arrows

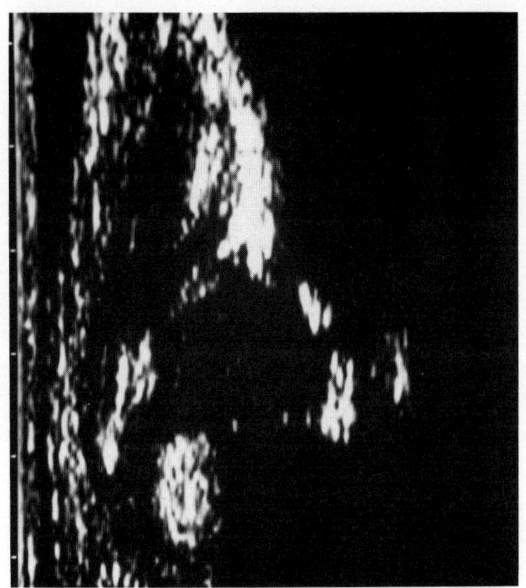

Fig. 14.32. P. A. eight weeks' old. Right hip joint. The bony formation is adequate. The cartilaginous acetabular roof is not widened but overlaps well. Hip joint corresponding to the child's age. Hip type IIa(+)

Fig. 14.33. The same patient as in Figure 14.32. Left hip joint eight weeks old. The bony formation is poor. The bony rim is grossly rounded or flattened. The cartilaginous acetabular roof is very wide and the acetabular labrum is compressed upwards. The cartilaginous structure is echo-poor. Hip type IIIa

14.6 Follow-up for progress in a type IIIa hip

A baby girl P. A. aged eight weeks was sent to our clinic for sonography for routine checkup after a breech delivery. The colleagues who referred her reported no positive clinical findings at the first examination but they asked for a prophylactic hip sonography because of the high risk of dysplasia. Sonographic findings on the right-hand side (Fig. 14.32) correspond to the child's age but on the left side there was a definite sonographic dislocation with an unambiguous sonographic instability (Fig. 14.33). Because of this instability, treatment with retention in a Fettweis plaster followed for a period of four weeks. At the end of this time clinical and sonographic stability had been achieved and further treatment was carried on with abduction in a Hilgenrein splint. At the checkup examination at the age of 4.5 months (that is, 2.5 months after the start of

therapy), the findings were almost symmetrical on both sides. On the previously healthy right side (Fig. 14.34) the bony formation is correct and the cartilaginous acetabular roof overlaps well. The femoral capital ossification centre was also visible. On the left, dislocated side, the findings were also completely normal for the child's age (Fig. 14.35).

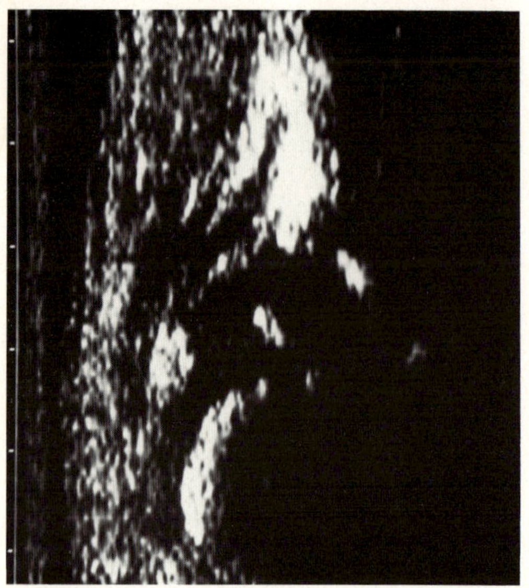

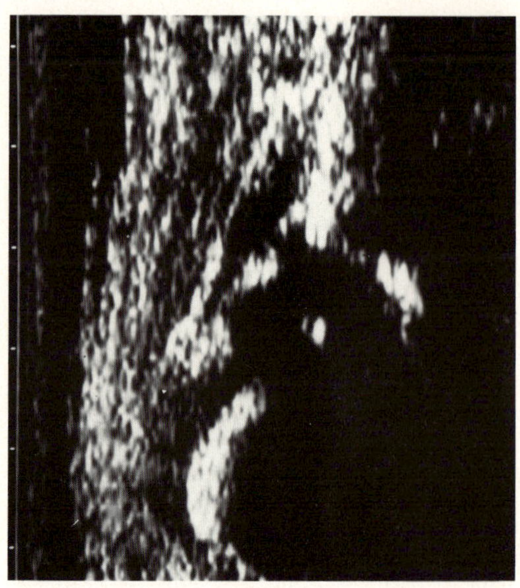

Fig. 14.34. P. A. 4.5 months old. Normal right hip joint for comparison with Figure 14.32. The bony formation is good, the bony rim is angulated, the cartilaginous acetabular roof sits on a wide base and is overlapping and the femoral capital ossification centre has appeared. Hip type I

Fig. 14.35. P. A. 4.5 months old. Left hip joint for comparison with the subluxed state shown in figure 14.33. The bony formation is now good and the bony rim is angulated. The cartilaginous acetabular roof is somewhat wide but clasps the femoral head well. Findings are commensurate for age: hip type I. In comparison with figure 15.34 (the normal right hip joint), the cartilaginous part of the roof appears somewhat wider and larger than it does on the healthy side

This chapter is aimed at improving familiarity with hip sonograph by giving further worked examples. The accompanying text has been deliberately kept short in order to make the findings clearer.

In order to increase the variety among the images, images are demonstrated taken with various apparatus and at various magnifications. The questions in the text have their answers in the legends to the figures.

Questions

Fig. 15.1
Does this sonogram fulfil the criteria for exact measurement technique?

Fig. 15.2
Seven month old hip joint. What type is it?

Fig. 15.3
Can you identify the anatomical structures on this image?

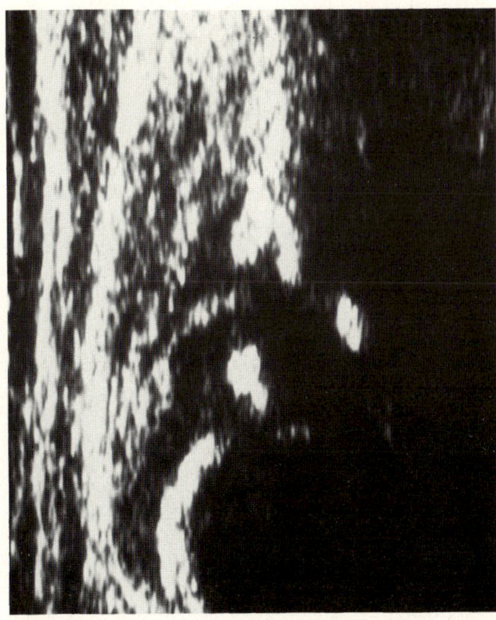

Fig. 15.1. This sonogram should not be used for measurement as the acetabular roof has been sectioned in a plane which lies too far dorsally and runs obviously over the concavity of the iliac wing (gluteal fossa)

Fig. 15.2. The bony formation is seriously deficient and the bony promontory is rather flat. The cartilaginous acetabular roof does not overlap the femoral head well. Classification according to this description leads to consideration of the hip joint in the borderline area of IIc and IIIa. The exact typing is given by the measurement technique. $\alpha = 47°$, $\beta = 70°$. Hip type IIc

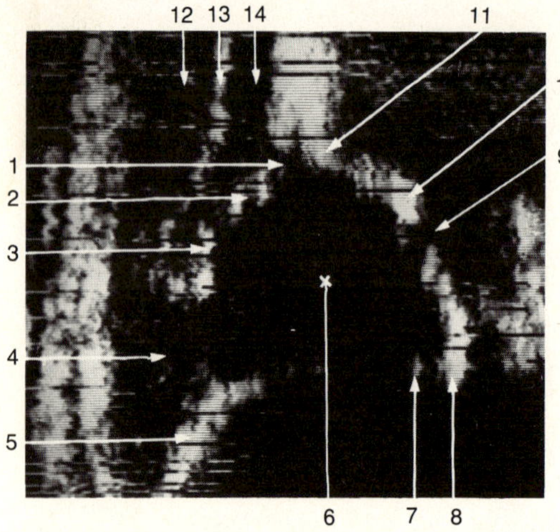

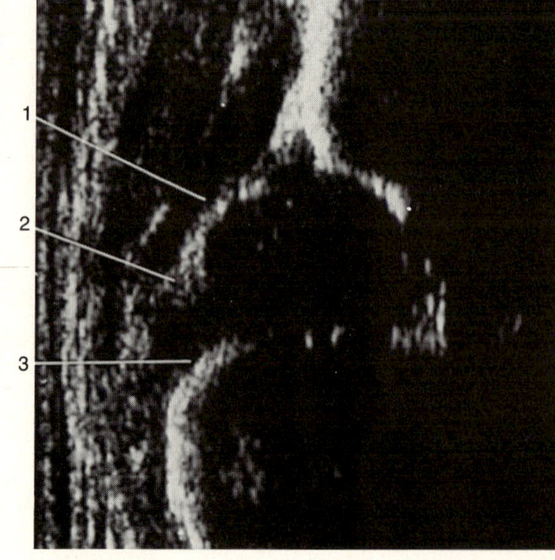

Fig. 15.3.
 1 Cartilaginous acetabular roof
 2 Acetabular labrum
 3 Joint capsule
 4 Greater trochanter
 5 Osteochondral junction
 6 Femoral head
 7 Ligament of the head of the femur
 8 Iliac bone
 9 Triradiate cartilage
10 Iliac bone
11 Bony promontory
12 & l4 Gluteal muscles
13 Intermuscular septum

Fig. 15.4.
1 Joint capsule
2 Folded area of joint capsule
3 Osteochondral junction

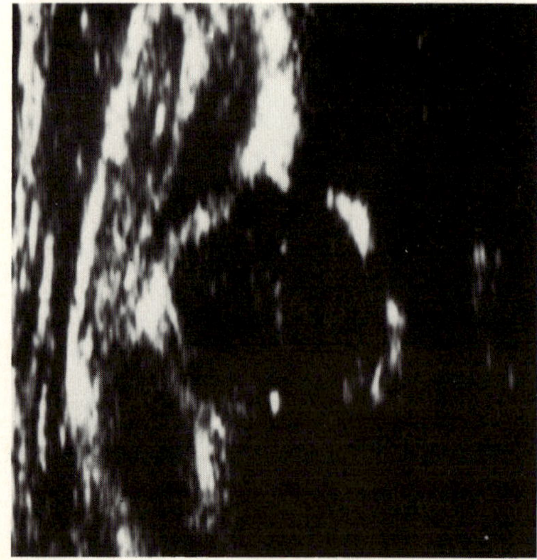

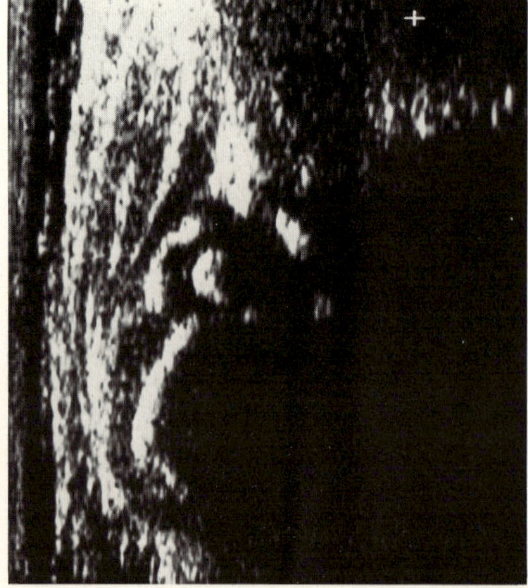

Fig. 15.5. Good bony formation, the bony promontory is well contoured, the cartilaginous promontory overlaps well. $\alpha = 60°$, $\beta = 70°$, type Ib. This hip must thus be considered to be completely matured

Fig. 15.6. The femoral head ossification centre should not be included in the diagnosis of dysplasia. A typical half moon phenomenon

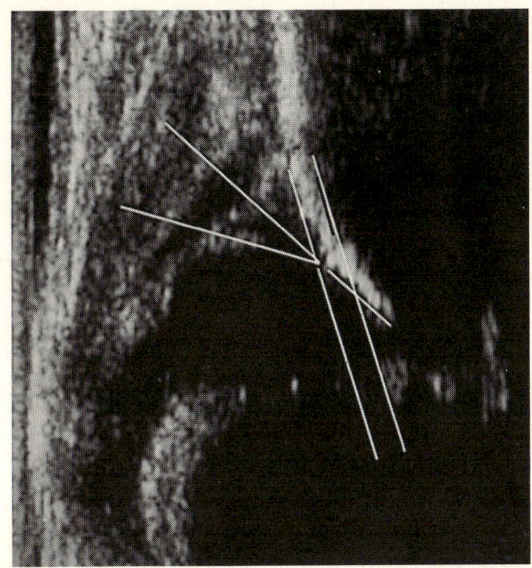

Fig. 15.7. Bony formation is deficient, the cartilaginous promontory is wide and compressed. The baseline and the accessory lines are drawn in.
$\alpha = 35°$, $\beta = 115°$, type IIIa

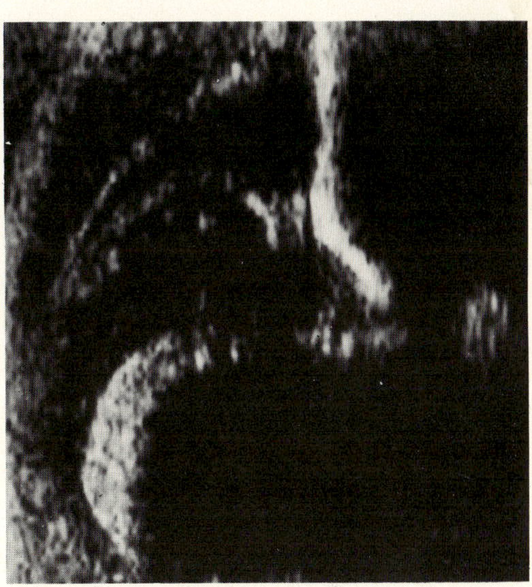

Fig. 15.8. The bony formation is poor, the bony promontory is flat. The femoral head is dislocated, and proximal to the femoral head the only thing that can be seen is the echo-poor zone of the gluteus minimus muscle. The cartilaginous roof is squashed between the femoral head and the true acetabulum. type IV joint

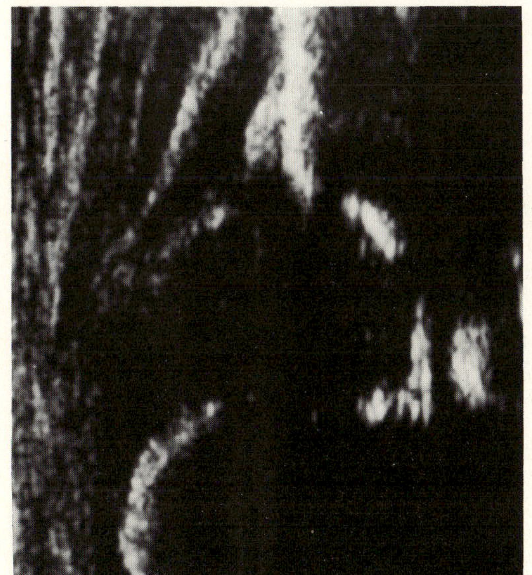

Fig. 15.9. Six week old hip joint. The bony formation is adequate. The bony promontory is round. The cartilaginous acetabular roof is widened, the femoral head is overlapped well and the ossification centre is absent. Type II

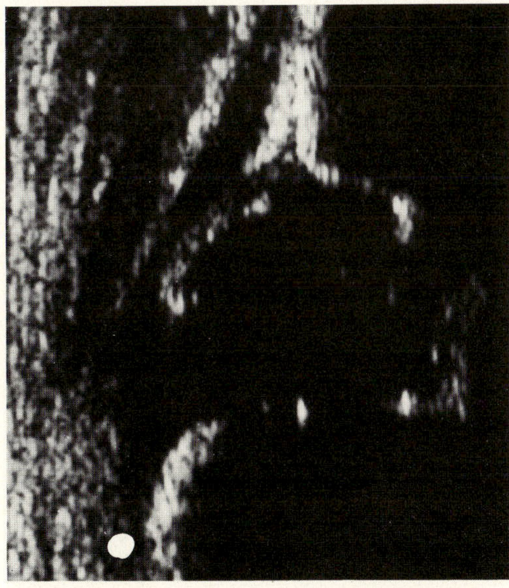

Fig. 15.10. Eight week old joint. The bony formation is good. The bony promontory is blunted. The cartilaginous acetabular roof overlaps the femoral head. The femoral capital ossification centre is absent. Type I

Fig. 15.4
On this hip, name the main anatomical parts. What type is it?

Fig. 15.5
Image of a neonatal hip. Does this hip correspond to the minimum acceptable degree of maturity?

Fig. 15.6
Here, the femoral capital ossification centre has been displaced laterally. Is the hip subluxed?

Fig. 15.7
Describe the findings in this hip.

Fig. 15.8
Image of a four week old baby. What hip type is present?

Fig. 15.9
Six week old hip joint. Describe the findings and give the hip type.

Fig. 15.10
An eight week old hip joint. Describe the findings and give the type.

Abduction of hip
  Relationship to dysplasia   98
Acetabulum
  Developmental anatomy   21
  Dysplasia   21, 23, 29
    Distinction from normal   92
    Prognosis   101, 103
    Relationship to risk factors   95
  Floor
    Layers   20, 35, 54
  Histology   23
  Labrum   20, 21
    Anatomical relations   34
    Definition of standard plane   57
    Displacement   21, 46
    Identification   61
  Limbus   34
  Rim
    Bony   37, 39
      Identification   61
    Cartilaginous
    Comparison with femoral head   49
      Echogenicity in   48
  Roof   32
    Bony
      Description   83, 84
        Cartilaginous   36, 41
      Developing echogenicity in   50
      Increased echogenicity   42
      Secondary ossification   52
    Compression   21, 83
    Degeneration   103
    Relationship to osteoarthrosis   71
    Variation in coverage   53
Angle
  Alpha   78, 83
    Accuracy of measurement   58
    Compared with radiographic acetabular angle   99
    Definition   61
    Relation to bony roofing   67
    Variation with age   69, 71, 101
  Beta   78
    Accuracy of measurement   58
    Relation to cartilaginous roof   67
Angles   84
Arthrography   17
Asymmetry of groin folds
  Relationship to dysplasia   98
Birth

Multiple
  Relationship to dysplasia   97
Breech presentation
  Relationship to dysplasia   96
    Comparison of flexed and extended types   96

Cartilage   17, 19, 20, 21, 23, 25, 28
  Histological structure   42
  See also Acetabular roof, cartilaginous
  Triradiate   20, 54
Computed tomography   18
Cradle   87
Critical range   73

Diagnosis
  Clinical
    'Silent' cases   17
Dislocation   74, 77
Dysplasia
  See Acetabulum, dysplasia

Echo gap   28, 29
  Perichondrium   33
Examination
  Clinical   87
    Relationship to dysplasia   97, 98
  Procedure   77
  Technique   87

Family history
  Relationship to dysplasia   96
Fascia
  Lunate   20, 54
Femur
  Capital epiphysis   31, 32, 56
    Ossification centre   19
  Head   28
    Anatomical relations   36, 37
    Reaction to pressure   44
  Neck   28, 30
Film
  Fluid   35
Fold
  Capsular   31
  Connective tissue   38

Half-moon phenomenon   32
Harcke
  Ultrasound technique   64

Hilgenrein line 32
Hip
 Dislocation 46
 Dysplasia
  See Acetabulum, dysplasia
 Positioning 17
 Type
  D 74
   Example 113
   Historical note 68
  I 39, 67
  Ia
   Distinction from type Ib 68
  Ib
   Comparison with type Ia 95
   Description 83
  II 40, 68
  IIa(+)
   Distinction from type IIa(−) in newborn 71
  IIb 72
  IIc 73
  III 41, 68, 74
   Distinction from type IV 47
   Transformation to type IV 78
  IIIa 42
   Distinction from type IIIb 50
  IIIa/IV Transitional 47
   Example 109, 111, 119
  IIIb 37, 42
   Example 115
   Prognosis 45
  IV 46, 68, 74
  Transitional form 68
  Variation with age 69, 72, 83
 Types
  Distribution in population 95
  Premature infants 73
Hypomochlion 21

Ilium
 Inferior border 54
  Appearance of 'tailoring' 59
 Wing 33, 56
  Recognition in abnormal hips 58
Image
 Projection 39
 Size 14, 15, 60
Impedance, acoustic 2

Joint capsule 21, 28, 31, 33, 46, 105, 106
Junction
 Osteochondral 19, 29, 30

Labrum
 See Acetabulum, labrum
Line
 Acetabular roof
  Definition 58
 Base
  Definition 59
  Accessory 60

Cartilaginous roof
 Definition 61
Lorenz
 Ultrasound technique 64

Magnetic resonance imaging 18
Maturation
 Acceptable rate 71
 Asymmetry of 5
Measurement
 Comparison of techniques 58

Neolimbus 21
 Ortolani sign 80
Neonates
 Treatment 107

Ortolani sign
 Relationship to ultrasound findings 80
 Sonographic equivalent 80
Ossification
 Delayed 41, 72
  Acetabular roof 103
 Early ultrasound appearance
  Acetabular roof 52
  Femoral head 31
 Physiological 52
 Seen at ultrasound 99, 100
Osteoarthrosis 71

Palisade, acoustic 30
Perichondrium 33, 37, 47
 Gap 33
Periosteum 33, 60
Piezo-electric effect 2, 3
Plane
 Coronal 27, 53
 Rotated 53
 Standard 8, 36
  Definition 54, 55, 57
   Dislocated joints 57
 Tilted 53
 Variation in 53
Position
 Of examiner 88–91
 Of infant 17, 63, 87–91
Prematurity
 Relationship to dysplasia 97
 Screening programmes 102
Probe
 Manipulation technique 91

Radiography 17
 Compared with ultrasound 99
 Indications 99
Roser-Ortolani sign
 See Ortolani sign

Screening 101, 102
Shadow, acoustic
 See Ultrasound, artefacts

Situation, standard   36
Soft tissues   27
Sonometer   67
Stability   73
  Definition   78
  Relationship to dysplasia   97

Tönnis
  Classification of subluxation
    Compared with hip types   100
  grades of dislocation   80
Treatment   103
  Aims   103–107
  Compliance   107
  Harness   103, 107
  Of neonates   107
  Overhead ('gallows') traction   104
  Phases   103–106
  Plaster   106
Trochater, greater   28

Ultrasound
  Age limits   108
  Artefacts   4, 11
    Acoustic shadow   4, 32, 60
    Reverberation   50
  Compared with radiography   99
  Compound scanner   4
  Controls   11, 12
  Fields   3, 10, 12
  Focal zone   3
  Frequency   2
  Hard copy   14, 15
  Historical   1
    locomotor system   1, 2
  Linear array   4, 7, 8
  Physical properties   2–5
  Placement of probe   9
  Safety   4, 5
  Scanning methods   4
  Sector scanner   4, 7, 8
  Technical requirements   8, 13
  Techniques
    Comparison of various   62–64
    Minimum standard examination   63
  Zoom   9